Paediatric Hip Disorders

The illustration on the binding
is used by kind permission of
Mercer Rang, Hospital for Sick Children,
Toronto, Canada

Paediatric Hip Disorders

EDITED BY

G. C. BENNET

FRCS

Consultant Orthopaedic Surgeon
Royal Hospital for Sick Children
Glasgow

BLACKWELL SCIENTIFIC PUBLICATIONS

OXFORD EDINBURGH LONDON

BOSTON PALO ALTO MELBOURNE

© 1987 by Blackwell Scientific Publications
Editorial Offices:
Osney Mead, Oxford, OX2 0EL
    (Orders: Tel. 0865 240201)
8 John Street, London, WC1N 2ES
23 Ainslie Place, Edinburgh, EH3 6AJ
52 Beacon Street, Boston
    Massachusetts 02108, USA
667 Lytton Avenue, Palto Alto
    California 94301, USA
107 Barry Street, Carlton
    Victoria 3053, Australia

First published 1987

Typeset by Morrison Reprographic Services,
Glasgow and printed and bound in Oxford by the
Alden Press.

DISTRIBUTORS

USA
    Year Book Medical Publishers
    35 East Wacker Drive
    Chicago, Illinois 60601
    (Orders: Tel. 312 726-9733)

Canada
    The C.V. Mosby Company
    5240 Finch Avenue East,
    Scarborough, Ontario
    (Orders: Tel. 416-298-1588)

Australia
    Blackwell Scientific Publications
        (Australia) Pty Ltd
    107 Barry Street
    Carlton, Victoria 3053
    (Orders: Tel. (03) 347 0300)

British Library
Cataloguing in Publication Data

Paediatric hip disorders.
    1. Hip Joint—Diseases 2. Pediatric orthopedia
    I. Bennet, G.C.
    617'.581 RJ482.H55

ISBN 0–632–01509–8

Contents

Contributors

G. C. BENNET *Consultant Orthopaedic Surgeon, Royal Hospital for Sick Children, Yorkhill, Glasgow.*

N. J. BLOCKEY *Consultant Orthopaedic Surgeon, Royal Hospital for Sick Children, Yorkhill, Glasgow.*

A. CATTERALL *Consultant Orthopaedic Surgeon, Children's Orthopaedic Unit, Royal National Orthopaedic Hospital, Stanmore.*

G. A. EVANS *Consultant Orthopaedic Surgeon, Children's Orthopaedic Unit, The Robert Jones and Agnes Hunt Orthopaedic Hospital, Oswestry.*

M. F. McNICOL *Consultant Orthopaedic Surgeon, Princess Margaret Rose Orthopaedic Hospital, Fairmilehead, Edinburgh.*

M. G. H. SMITH *Consultant Orthopaedic Surgeon, Royal Hospital for Sick Children, Yorkhill, Glasgow.*

I. G. STOTHER *Consultant Orthopaedic Surgeon, Stobhill General Hospital and the Royal Infirmary, Glasgow.*

I. P. TORODE *Consultant Orthopaedic Surgeon, Royal Melbourne Children's Hospital, Parkville, Australia.*

Preface

Hip disorders in childhood is a topic guaranteed to generate debate amongst paediatric orthopaedic surgeons. Such argument is often undertaken from deeply entrenched and publicly know positions. That there is so much disagreement may be explained in many cases by a lack of hard data upon which to base a convincing case. In this field, perhaps more than in any other in orthopaedics, the aphorism 'to be unsure is uncomfortable, to be certain, ridiculous', should be remembered. Whilst such debate is often stimulating for the participants, it inevitably leads to confusion in the mind of the trainee surgeon or the more established orthopaedic surgeon who makes only occasional forays into this field. It is to this audience that the book is addressed.

The book provides a sound basis for the management of the more common hip conditions of childhood and some guidance for those seen less often. The common theme running through the book is the necessity to treat a child safely and, often of the basis of inadequate information, to anticipate the likely result of any surgical intervention many years ahead. There is no denying that this is a difficult task.

That said, however, this is a fascinating field and one in which there is great potential for restoring normal function to a crippled child. The rewards of successful treatment are great for both the child and the surgeon.

Finally, attention must be paid to the child and family as well as to the disease. This has been summarized by Dr Robert Salter as 'we must treat the child's head as well as the femoral head'. This is sound advice.

1

Development of the Hip

G. C. BENNET

Normal development

Good paediatric practice is based upon knowledge of the natural history of disease and its effects, not only in childhood, but also in adult life. One must aim to anticipate the outcome of a pathological process and, on that basis, make therapeutic decisions. Prediction of the abnormal is obviously dependent upon a knowledge of the normal so that the starting point in the consideration of any aspect of children's orthopaedics is that of the growth and development of the part. The starting point in the study of childhood hip disorders is therefore the pre- and early postnatal development of the hip. Only with such knowledge can, for example, the genesis of congenital disorders or the effects of vascular impairment on the growth of the hip be understood. This chapter does not aim to be scholarly but rather a practical guide derived from published work on the topic.

Development of the human form is divided into several stages. The first two weeks after implantation is known as the *ovular stage* which is in turn succeeded by the *embryonic period*. During this time the bones and joints develop to an extent that, by the end of this stage at around 8 weeks, they resemble those of a miniature adult. In other words complete differentiation has taken place. In the context of the hip, the joint is fully formed and a circulation is established. Such complete differentiation marks the end of the embryonic period. Before then, if an abnormality of development occurs it is termed an *embryopathy*. This is a true structural malformation, for example proximal focal femoral deficiency.

There then follows a period of growth, that is an increase in cellular size and number, in the already differentiated structures. This is the *fetal period* which stretches from the end of the embryonic period to the time of birth. An abnormality arising during this time is termed a *fetopathy*. By definition it is an abnormality of an initially normally formed part and unlike an embryopathy, is potentially reversible. To emphasize that growth does not change dramatically immediately after birth, the fetal period is often combined with the first month after life, the neonatal period, and collectively termed the *perinatal period*. During the discussion that follows, reference will be made to prenatal development at certain times.

Normally such fetal development is signified by the measurement of the crown–rump length and whilst this obviously may vary somewhat between fetuses of the same age, it does give some guide to the state of development reached.

All bones in the fetal skeleton are formed on a mesenchymal scaffold. Some ossify directly on this template, specifically the bones of the skull and the clavicles, these being examples of intramembranous ossification. Elsewhere the mesenchymal model first changes to cartilage and subsequently calcifies and ossifies. This represents enchondral ossification and is the method of formation of the femur and pelvic bones. Whilst the mechanics are slightly different, the bone formed by both methods is identical.

The ultimate shape of a bone is determined to a large extent by factors intrinsic to the cells which form the final structure, environmental factors being of only secondary importance.

In very early stages of development the embryo is made up of two layers, the endoderm and the ectoderm. Soon a third layer, the mesoderm, appears and invaginates between the other two. It is from this that the skeleton and associated soft tissues will develop. At around 4 weeks post ovulation, that is 4–5 mm crown–rump stage, two small proturberances, the limb buds, appear on the ventrolateral

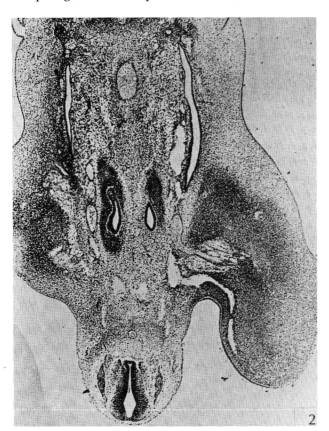

Fig. 1.1 10 mm embryo (x22HE). Limb bud formation. The blastema of the hip is homogeneous and the muscular and osseous primordia cannot be separately distinguished. (Reproduced with permission from Strayer L. 1971 Embryology of the human hip joint. *Clinical Orthopaedics and Related Research,* **74,** 223.)

aspect of the embryo (Fig.1.1). Similar protruberances appear for the upper limb, these usually being slightly in advance of the lower. Within a few days of their formation a blood supply, in the form of a capillary plexus, is present.

At the apex of the limb buds, the mesenchyme is in close contact with the overlying ectoderm. This ectoderm, at the leading edge of the bud, differentiates to form the apical ectodermal ridge (AER) which is a specialized area responsible for 'pulling out' the limb and inducing the underlying mesenchyme to differentiate in a proximodistal sequence. Whilst the ectoderm ultimately gives rise to skin, the mesoderm develops into three layers each of which in turn develops into differing parts of the limb. The superficial layer, lying immediately beneath the AER, is a region of marked cellular activity which gives rise to the remaining two zones namely the intermediate, from which the skeletal musculature and certain paraskeletal structures namely periosteum, perichondrium and joint capsules will develop and the deep layer from which the primitive skeleton takes origin. In the area of the deep layer of the mesenchyme, the cells multiply and become densely packed at the site of ultimate bone information. This, the skeletal blastema, forms a rough outline of the future bone. By 5–6 weeks' gestation or 10 mm crown–rump stage, the form of the skeleton is usually distinguishable. As the blastema matures by the transformation of mesenchymal cells into chondrocytes, the mesenchyme surrounding the cartilage model becomes compressed to form an enveloping membrane called the perichondrium. This has two layers; an inner chondrogenic responsible for appositional growth of the model and an outer fibrous one which functions as a limiting membrane.

The whole model does not develop at the same pace. Thus, whilst one area, for example the trochanter, is in the precartilagenous blastemal stage, another, perhaps the distal end of the femur, is in the form of cartilage model whilst a third, the diaphysis, is already formed of fetal bone. Chondrification of the femoral model, which commences at about 6 weeks, starts centrally and extends towards the ends. Cell division takes place predominantly at the ends of the model so that the cells of the central diaphysis are the oldest and thus have time to mature (Fig. 1.2). These cells enlarge and become separated as they secrete cartilage martix which ultimately calcifies. This prevents diffusion of nutrients to the contained cartilage cells resulting in cell death. At about the seventh week of intrauterine life, formation of the primary ossification centre commences (Fig. 1.3). Around the central area of mature or dead cartilage cells, the perichondrium is invaded by blood vessels. This stimulates the differentiation of the cells in the chondrogenic layer into osteoblasts and these in turn lay down osteoid tissue which is quickly mineralized and forms the primary bone collar. The membrane surrounding the bone is now periosteum albeit still in continuity with perichondrium both proximally and distally. As the collar matures and more layers of osteoid are laid down, the dead cartilage cells are invaded by a bud of capillaries and osteogenic cells derived from the periosteum which breaks down the calcified cartilage at the middle of the model. Bone is then laid down on the remaining bits of cartilage, an example of

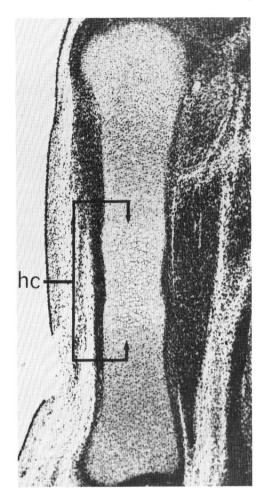

Fig. 1.2 Low power view of part of a leg of a rabbit embryo. Note the hypertrophied cartilage cells (HC) in the diaphysis. (Reproduced with permission from Ham and Cormack 1979 *Histophysiology of Cartilage, Bones and Joints,* p.423, J. B. Lippincott, Philadelphia.)

enchondral ossification. The primary centre of ossification has then been formed. Whilst only the femur is considered here, a similar process is happening in all the long bones of the body at around the same time. One of the vessels contained in the periosteal bud, which enters at the distal portion of the middle third of the bone, will ultimately become the nutrient artery. Bone formation spreads out from the primary ossification centre with cartilage destruction followed by enchondral ossification extending towards each end of the bone, this advance being paralleled by appositional growth, originating from the periosteum, the latter always slightly preceding the former. By the end of the embryonic period, the primary bone collar extends over about 20% of the shaft of the femur (Gardner 1972). By term, 80% will be ossified, the rest still being in the cartilage stage (Gardner & Gray 1970).

Once the femur has adequate structural support provided by subperiosteal bone, the cancellous bone in the centre in the centre of the shaft is resorbed and myeloid tissue, originating from the periosteal bud, replaces it so that, by about

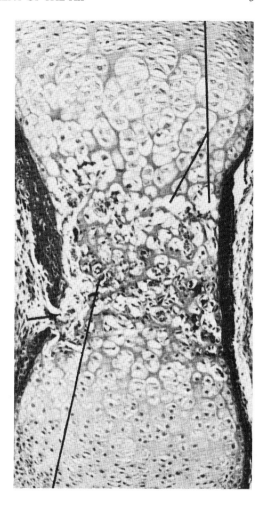

Fig. 1.3 Formation of primary ossification centre (metaphysis of mouse embryo). Periosteal bud (arrow) marks the ingrowth of osteogenic cells and blood vessels. (Reproduced with permission from Ham and Cormack 1979 *Histophysiology of Cartilage, Bones and Joints*, J. B. Lippincott, Philadelphia.)

the fourth month of intrauterine life, a central marrow cavity will have formed (Ham & Cormack 1979).

Development of the pelvic bones proceeds along similar lines. In the blastemal stage the mesenchymal models of the innominate bone and that of the femur are in continuity. Both then go through the stages of chondrification and ossification, the femur always being a little more advanced. The outline of the pelvic bones is present in the blastemal stage in the 10 mm embryo and all three begin to chondrify in the embryonic period. The ilium is the first to ossify. Although it may commence in the embryonic period, it more usually occurs at around the third month when an area just above the greater sciatic notch develops as the primary ossification centre.

Just as in the femur, the cells in this region hypertrophy. The perichondrium on the inner and outer tables of the bone are then subject to vascular invasion forming periosteum which in turn lays down a primary bone collar. Once again, invasion by a periosteal bud takes place and the primary ossification centre is formed by the replacement of degenerate cartilage. Further ossification spreads in three directions: the posterior and caudal projections are obvious by the third month whereas the anterior usually does not make its appearance until the fourth (Gardner 1972). By term, most of the ilium is ossified. The ischium and pubis both ossify in a similar manner, the former in the fourth month and the latter in the fifth. Ossification in all these bones converges and meets at the Y-shaped triradiate cartilage, the ilium facing the superior aspect, the ischium the posterior and the pubis the anterior. Subsequent growth of all three takes place in an interrelated way so as to accommodate the expanding femoral head.

Whilst this is proceeding, the hip joint is developing rapidly. As we have already noted, in blastemal form, the femur and pelvic bones are in continuity. As they develop, an area of unchondrified blastema remains between the chondrified elements of the skeletal analage. This marks the site of the future hip joint (Fig. 1.4). At the 15 mm crown–rump stage, the outline of an area of diminished density

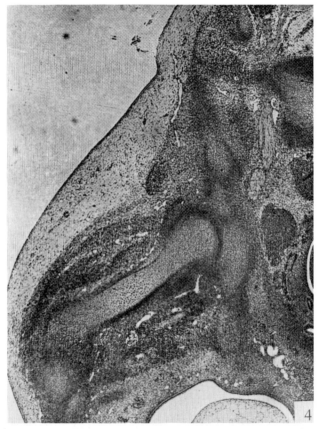

Fig. 1.4 17.5 mm embryo (x22HE). The outline of the future joint is marked by the darkly staining cells. The elements of the innominate primordia can be seen. (Reproduced with permission from Strayer L. 1971 Embryology of the human hip joint. *Clinical Orthopaedics and Related Research,* **74,** 225.)

is present where the hip joint will form. Soon it is compacted and becomes a region of increased, rather than diminished, density. Initially it is homogeneous but, by

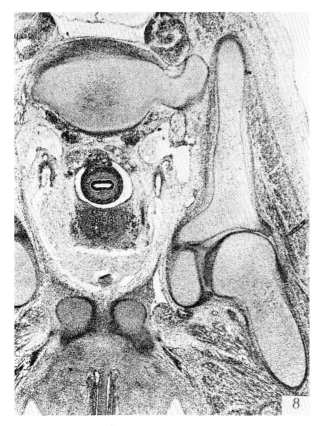

Fig. 1.5 30 mm embryo (x22HE). The ligamentum teres can be seen as a line of darkly stained cells. The labrum and its relationship to the capsule can also be seen (Reproduced with permission from Strayer L. 1971 Embryology of the Human Hip *Clinical Orthopaedics and Related Research*, **74**, 229.)

the seventh week, three layers are evident. On the outer layers of the sandwich are two chondrogenic regions continuous with the perichondrium of the innominate and femoral models whilst between them is a less dense region of loosely packed cells, the interzone, continuous at the periphery with the synovial mesenchyme (Wheeler Haines 1981).

   The chondrogenic layers will form the articular cartilage of the acetabulum and femur whereas the central zone will undergo autolytic degeneration. When the joint makes its first appearance it subtends an arc of only around 65–70° (Strayer 1971). This ultimately deepens to 180°, a process dependent upon there being normal function in the surrounding muscles and, presumably, mechanical pressure from the femoral head. Only when the depression forms a full semicircle does cavitation commence, usually at about the eighth week or 20 mm crown–rump stage (Gardner & Gray 1970). The process starts at the periphery with appearance of small spaces in the intermediate zone. These coalesce and spread towards the central part of the depression such that, by 10 weeks, a recognizable joint cavity is present which almost completely encloses the femoral head.

The ligamentum teres forms *in situ*. It is can be seen at 7 weeks as a collection of primitive fibroblasts aligned in the axis of the femur (Fig. 1.5), crossing the presumptive joint space. Cavitation then takes place around it such that, by the 30 mm stage, it is well defined. The transverse acetabular ligament and the labrum are similarly formed and become defined by cavitation taking place around them. The synovial membrane is first evident shortly after cavitation although, at that stage, it is difficult to distinguish the layer of cells that will form the synovium from those that give rise to the capsule. By around the ninth week, blood vessels are present in the synovial cells. Immediately superficial to the synovial membrane is the joint capsule, this being a direct continuation of the perichondrium of the femur distally, blending into a cellular layer overlying proximally the labrum (Gardner & Gray 1980). Following cavitation of the joint space, collagen is deposited in the capsule, such that, by 50 mm crown–rump that is around 11 weeks, it can be seen as a discrete structure. Over the ensuing weeks, further collagen is laid down in certain areas of the capsule to form the intrinsic ligaments (Gardner & Gray 1950).

By the same time, the hip joint has developed to the point that there is a fully formed joint cavity containing differentiated articular cartilage and a spherical head some 2 mm in diameter. As the neck is short, the capsule, which inserts along the intertrochanteric line, contains only the head.

With further development the hip joint becomes shallower. Initially almost the whole head is contained with the acetabulum but with subsequent growth and increasing movement, the amount of head cover diminishes. In other words, stability has been sacrificed for movement. This is most obvious at the time of birth when the acetebulum may form only one third of a sphere. As the head at this time is hemispherical, its maximum diameter is not contained within the joint (Ralis & McKibben 1973). This is the time of maximum instability.

Throughout pre- and postnatal life, changes take place in both the angle of anteversion of the neck and the neck shaft angle. In the first half of fetal life, anteversion is extremely variable and, whilst difficult to measure accurately in the fetus because of the shortness of the femoral neck, may certainly be negative in the early stages of development (Wantanabe 1974). Torsion alters this and it soon becomes positive, by term exceeding adult values (Stanislavjevic 1964). Acetabular anteversion is also variable, averaging around 7° at birth (McKibben 1970). Little correlation has been found between the degree of anteversion of the femur and that of the acetabulum, a wide range of each still being compatible with joint stability (McKibben 1970). The neck-shaft angle in the neonate at around 135°–145°, is somewhat greater than that found in adult life when 125° is a more usual value (Stanislavjevic 1964).

The most momentous changes in the postnatal period are the development of the femoral neck and the formation of a secondary ossific nucleus within the chondroepiphysis. The latter usually takes place 4–6 months postnatally. Its development is dependent upon normal biomechanical stresses being applied to the femoral head, as is evidenced by its late appearance in a dysplastic or dislocated hip. The ossification centre develops in much the same way as has already been described with respect to the primary centre namely initial hypertrophy of the cartilage cells followed by their calcification and ossification. In subsequent months enlargement occurs centripitally with flattening where it comes into contact with the physis to produce the final hemispherical shape. Between the ages of three and four years, the greater trochanter forms its ossific nucleus. Occasionally a second may develop over the next couple of years but this usually rapidly fuses with the primary centre (Ogden 1983).

Femoral neck growth plate

The function of the growth plate is to provide for longitudinal and latitudinal

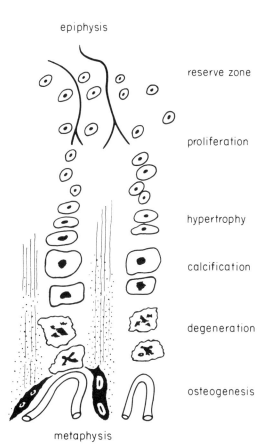

epiphysis

reserve zone

proliferation

hypertrophy

calcification

degeneration

osteogenesis

Fig. 1.6 The structure of the growth plate.

metaphysis

growth of the bone. It develops between the primary and secondary ossification centres of the femur. Whilst its shape changes from planar to dome-shaped during growth, its internal architecture alters little, the various zones mirroring the differing functions of each region (Fig. 1.6). The cartilagenous zone can be divided into the following areas:

The reserve or resting zone

This is located immediately beneath the epiphysis. Here cells are few, but matrix is abundant. The likeliest function of this region is the production and storage of nutritional materials for use in other zones.

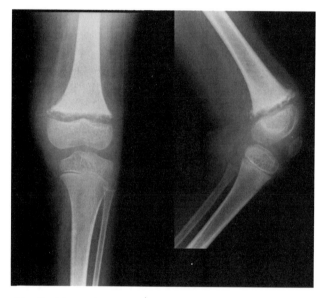

Fig. 1.7 Widening of the distal femoral growth plate in a child with myelomeningocele, presumably due to repeated minor trauma.

The proliferative zone

This is a metabolically active area which has a blood supply and where aerobic metabolism takes place. The cells at the top of the column are actively dividing and can be regarded as the germinal cells of the epiphyseal plate. With division the chondrocytes become aligned vertically in palisades and collagen is laid down between the cell columns forming longditudinal intercolumnar septa. The rate of growth of a bone is obviously directly related to the rate of cellular division in this region. To avoid the plate progressively increasing in width, the rate of new cell formation must be matched by an identical rate of osseous transformation in the metaphyseal region. Occasionally this mechanism fails and widening of the plate results (Fig. 1.7).

Hypertrophic zone

This is an avascular zone where anaerobic metabolism occurs. Proximally the cells enlarge considerably but, by the bottom, nuclear fragmentation and cell death has taken place. This is presumably due to depletion of glycogen within the cells. As the cells move through the zone, calcium is progressively released. As calcium accumulation within the mitochondria is an active process, its release, which results in calcification of the matrix, can be related to the coincidental depletion of glycogen (Bighton 1983).

Zone of transformation

Here the intercolumnar matrix is calcified to form the primary spongiosum. This zone therefore consists of vascularized calcified cartilage. Not until a little way down do osteoblasts begin to lay down bone by enchondral ossification. The more distal one goes, the more formed the bone becomes, passing through secondary spongiosum to lamellar bone.

Surrounding the physis are the fibrous groove of Ranvier and the perichondrial ring of Lacroix. The zone of Ranvier is the area of specialized cells located at the periphery of the plate which is the source of supply of chondrocytes to the plate thus providing a mechanism for its growth in diameter. The osseous ring of Lacroix is a proximal extension of the cortex of the metaphysis and acts as a limiting structure to the cells of the physis, at the same time providing mechanical support.

Each zone in the epiphyseal plate has a discrete blood supply. Vessels arising from the ascending cervical branches of the medial and lateral circumflex arteries pass through the resting zone to the area of cell division in the proliferative zone. Although they pass through the reserve zone, the low PO_2 in this region suggests that they do not actually supply it (Bighton 1983). Instead the supply is to the proliferative zone where a high PO_2 is found. These vessels terminate there and none pass through to the area of hypertrophic cells. At the distal end of the plate, the metaphysis has a plentiful blood supply derived in part from the metaphyseal branches of the ascending cervical arteries but predominantly from the nutrient artery of the femur which contributes some 80% of the total (Bighton 1983). These vessels take the form of loops and turn just at the base of the plate. No vessels pass from the metaphysis to the hypertrophic zone.

Development of the femoral neck in the postnatal period is dependent upon differing rates of growth within the proximal femoral growth plate which are in turn dictated by biomechanical stresses. At birth the growth plate is transversely orientated. As a consequence of the shortness of the neck only a small part of the medial metaphysis is intracapsular. The central part of the growth plate has a growth velocity greater than that on the medial side which itself has a velocity greater than the lateral portion (Ogden 1983). Thus more growth occurs centrally and medially and less on the lateral side and in the greater trochanter. This has two consequences: the femoral neck elongates and the capital femur moves proximally with respect to the greater trochanter, that is a positive articulotrochanteric distance (ATD) develops. As trochanteric growth is independent of that of the femur, if for any reason growth in the femoral neck is interrupted, trochanteric overgrowth and reversal of the ATD will occur. An example of this is to be found in avascular necrosis following treatment of congenital dislocation of the hip. Conversely, relative overgrowth on the medial side is evidenced by an increased neck shaft angle and an increased ATD. This can be found, for example in myelomeningocele where paralysis of the abductors reduces the stimulus to trochanteric growth.

Circulation of the hip

The pattern of blood supply to the developing hip changes quite dramatically between the neonatal period and infancy. These changes are of some importance in the genesis of abnormalities of the hip which may develop in early life.

Embryonic blood supply

Within a few days of the appearance of the limb bud in the embryo, a circulation is established within it. Initially there are several segmental vessels supplying the bud but one soon takes on a dominant role to become the stem artery, whilst the remainder form the collateral circulation. In the lower limb the original stem artery is ultimately of secondary importance, becoming the inferior gluteal whilst the femoral arteries bypass it to form the main vessels of supply (Ogden 1974).

Vessels first enter the shaft of the femur at the diaphysis following the development of the primary bone collar. There are usually several within the periosteal bud which is responsible for the formation of the primary ossific nucleus. Once again, one becomes dominant, this time becoming the nutrient artery. By about 11 weeks blood vessels derived from the epiphyseal arteries penetrate the femoral head at regular intervals around the capsular insertion. These course through the femoral head encased in cartilage canals which supply discrete regions, there being very little overlap in their areas of distribution. Although some of the nutritional requirements of the hyaline cartilage of the chondro-epiphysis are met by diffusion, an intrinsic supply is still essential. By the 85–95 mm stage there is a blood supply within the ligamentum teres. These vessels however, do not play a significant role in the supply of the femoral head as most terminate either within the ligament itself or superficially in the fovea. By the end of the embryonic period the basic pattern of the extra capsular blood supply is established and this same pattern persists throughout fetal and postnatal life. This contrasts with that of the intracapsular blood supply which changes significantly with growth.

Extracapsular blood supply

Two vessels contribute to the extra capsular blood supply: the medial and the lateral circumflex arteries (Fig. 1.8). Whilst the medial circumflex most commonly arises from the femoral artery, the lateral usually takes origin from the profunda femoris (Chung 1981). Both vessels arise at the level of the tendinous portion of the psoas just proximal to the lesser trochanter. From its origin the medial circumflex runs posteriorly between the tendon of the psoas and the adductor muscles. It continues as the transverse branch reaching the femur distal to the insertion of the hip joint capsule just superior to the lesser trochanter. It then runs on the posterior intertrochanteric line towards the trochanteric fossa.

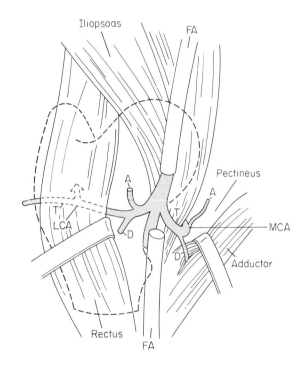

Fig. 1.8 The initial course of the extracapsular blood supply to the hip. The medial circumflex artery (MCA) and the lateral circumflex artery (LCA) are shown arising from the profunda femoris. Each divides into ascending (A), descending (D) and transverse (T) branches. The subsequent course of the transverse branches is described in the text. Reproduced with permission from J. A. Ogden 1982 in *Congenital Dislocation of the Hip* (Ed. M. O. Tachdjian) Churchill Livingstone, New York.

The lateral circumflex artery takes origin at the same level. Passing anterior to the psoas tendon it too gives off muscular branches before going between the branches of the femoral nerve to reach the anterior aspect of the femur where it runs deep to the rectus femoris, in close apposition to the bone, towards the trochanteric fossa. The medial and lateral circumflex arteries thus form a ring around the femoral neck with the medial supplying the posterior and lateral parts and the lateral the anterior. Although they both terminate in the trochanteric fossa they do not invariably anastomose with each other. Indeed Chung (1976) found that this basal or intertrochanteric anastomosis was complete in only 2 of 26 specimens. This pattern, established in early prenatal life, persists in the adult. The two circumflex arteries supply roughly equal portions of the trochanter where the multiple vessel system remains constant. Although the extracapsular course of the arteries persists, the development of the femoral neck leads to changes in the intracapsular supply. Initially multiple vessels arise from the extracapsular ring and gain access to the epiphyseal cartilage at the intertrochanteric line where the capsule in inserted. As there is little femoral neck, these vessels have no significant intracapsular course.

Intracapsular circulation

At birth, vessels penetrate the chondro-epiphysis every few millimetres along the capsular insertion, both anteriorly and posteriorly. Then, the circulation of the chondroepiphysis is divided roughly in half with the medial circumflex supplying the posterior aspect and the lateral the anterior. The same division of circulation to the trochanter and growth plate is also present. Whilst the growth plate itself is not penetrated by blood vessels some from each side run through the perichondral fibrocartilagenous complex to anastomose with each other. This means that a communication exists between the metaphyseal and epiphyseal circulations which may be of significance in the spread of infection. By the second year of life this anastomosis is insignificant. In the neonate there is an artery within the ligamentum teres, but it is of little functional importance in the development of the chondroepiphysis. Only after the age of 10 does the artery play a significant role in the circulation of the femoral head.

At birth, vessels can enter the epiphyseal hyaline cartilage without having a significant intracapsular course. This changes with the development of the femoral neck. As the neck elongates, the vessels within the capsule progressively coalesce such that, instead of there being a multiple vessel supply, the circulation of the chondroepiphysis comes to rely on a few. In place of vessels entering every few millimetres, the posterosuperior and posteroinferior cervical branches of the medial circumflex become almost the only vessels of supply (Fig. 1.9). Whilst coalition occurs in the intracapsular course the intraepiphyseal vessels remain multiple and arborized although persisting as end arteries. Both the posterosuperior and posteroinferior branches of the medial circumflex run beneath the synovial membrane forming a subsynovial anastomosis which also receives contributions from the lateral circumflex. The posteroinferior vessels normally run to their insertion on the epiphyseal side of the physis in a loose fold or retinacular reflection of the synovium. In contrast the posterosuperior arteries may run in grooves, covered with synovium, on the femoral neck or indeed may run within the cartilage itself (Ogden 1982). Either way this group of vessels is much more fixed in position.

Thus with the growth of the femoral neck, two primary circulatory systems

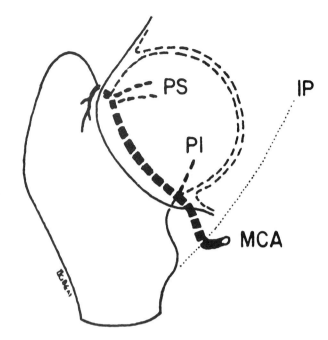

Fig. 1.9 The course of the medial circumflex artery (MCA). The predominant posterosuperior (PS) and posteroinferior (PI) branches are shown. (Reproduced with permission from J. A. Ogden 1982 In *Congenital Dislocation of the Hip*. (Ed. M. O. Tachdjian) Churchill Livingstone, New York.)

develop, each arising from the medial circumflex artery. The posteroinferior vessels distribute to the inferiomedial segment of the epiphysis and the medial aspect of the proximal part of the growth plate. The posterosuperior vessel accounts for the remaining areas and is therefore the dominant artery of supply. Changes are also taking place anteriorly (Fig. 1.10). As the neck develops and the anterior part of the articular surface overlaps it, fewer and fewer branches of the lateral circumflex artery are able to reach the chondroepiphysis. In consequence, they become the source of supply to the anterior metaphysis.

There are several anastomoses present in the region of the proximal femur, usually more of anatomical than practical interest as it is seldom that one source of supply can take over the territory of another in the event of an acute interruption of the usual blood supply. On the surface of the femoral neck, the subsynovial anastomosis gains its maximum contributions from the posterosuperior and inferior branches of the circumflex arteries. In the extra capsular region, as already noted, there is a variable anastomosis between the medial and lateral circumflex arteries in the intertrochanteric notch. This hardly changes with further development. A further anastomosis only develops once the ossific nucleus is present. Before its appearance there is a congregation of cartilage canals in the region where it will arise, these containing vessels mainly arising from the posterosuperior branches of the medial circumflex artery. Some, however, take origin from the posteroinferior branch so that, in the region of the ossific nucleus, a cross over between the two systems exists.

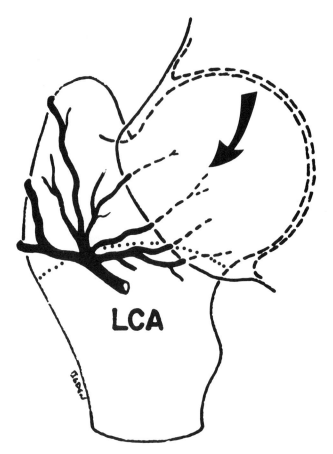

Fig. 1.10 The course of the lateral circumflex artery (LCA) in the infant. Whilst most of the supply is to the greater trochanter, intracapsular branches (arrow) supply part of the anterior chondro epiphysis. (Reproduced with permission from J. A. Ogden 1982 In *Congenital Dislocation of the Hip* (Ed. M. O. Tachdjian) Churchill Livingstone, New York.)

Avascular necrosis

Unlike other epiphyses, that of the proximal femur is always at risk from interruption of the blood supply. This is explained both by the development of a system based on a few, rather than many vessels, and the lack of adequate anastomoses.

In the young child, because of the presence of multiple vessels of supply within the capsule, any interruption which leads to appreciable changes within the epiphysis, must have occured in the extra capsular course of those vessels. Because of its longer and rather more tortuous course, the medial circumflex is more liable to interruption, usually by compression at specific points, than the lateral. Immobilization of the hip in the treatment of congenital dislocation of the hip is the most common cause for the development of avascular necrosis. Positioning in abduction and internal rotation may cause compression of the medial circumflex artery between the psoas and adductor muscles whilst the frog position may compress the posterosuperior branch of the medial circumflex artery against the brim of the acetabulum as it runs in the acetabular fossa. Surgery too can cause trouble, particularly damage to the medial circumflex artery during reduction of the hip by a medial approach. The lateral circumflex artery is much less likely to be damaged. Usually it is spared resulting in trochanteric overgrowth.

References

Bighton K. (1983) In *Management of Hip Disorders in Children* (Eds. J. F. Katz & R. S. Siffert) pp.51–69. J. B. Lippincott Co, Philadelphia.

Chung S. M. K. (1976) The arterial supply to the developing end of the human femur. *Journal of Bone and Joint Surgery,* **58A,** 961–70.

Chung S. M. K. (1981) *Hip Disorders in Infants and Children,* p.25. Lee & Feabiger, Philadelphia.

Gardner E. (1972) Prenatal development of the human hip joint, femur and hip bone. *American Association of Orthopaedic Surgeons Instructional Course Lectures,* **21,** 138–53.

Gardner E. & Gray D. J. (1950) Prenatal development of the human hip joint. *American Journal of Anatomy,* **87,** 163–211.

Gardner E. & Gray D. J. (1970) The prenatal development of the human femur. *American Journal of Anatomy,* **129,** 121–40.

Ham A. W. & Cormack D. H. (1979) *Histophysiology of Bone, Cartilage and Joints,* p.425. J. B. Lippincott, Toronto.

McKibben B. K. (1970) Anatomical factors in the stability of the hip in the newborn. *Journal of Bone and Joint Surgery,* **52B,** 148–59.

Ogden J. A. (1974) Changing patterns of proximal femoral vascularity. *Journal of Bone and Joint Surgery,* **56A,** 941–50.

Ogden J. A. (1982) In *Congenital Dislocation of the Hip* (Ed. M. O. Tachdjian) p.69. Churchill Livingstone, New York.

Ogden J. A. (1983) In *Management of Hip Disorders in Children* (Eds. J. F. Katz & R. S. Siffert) pp.1–32. J. B. Lippincott Co, Philadelphia.

Ralis Z. & McKibben B. (1973) Changes in shape of the human hip joint during its development; their relationship to its stability. *Journal of Bone and Joint Surgery,* **55B,** 780–5.

Stanislavjevic S. (1964) *Diagnosis and Treatment of Congenital Hip Pathology in the Newborn.* Williams and Wilkins Co., Baltimore.

Strayer L. M. (1971) Embryology of the human hip joint. *Clinical Orthopaedics and Related Research,* **74,** 221–40.

Watanabe R. S. (1974) Embryology of the human hip. *Clinical Orthopaedics and Related Research,* **98,** 8–26.

Wheeler-Haines R. (1947) The development of joints. *Journal of Anatomy,* **81,** 33–55.

Recommended reading

A. W. Ham & D. H. Cormack (1979) *Histophysiology of Cartilage Bone and Joints* J. B. Lippincott, Philadelphia.

Management of Hip Disorders in Children J. F. Katz & R. S. Siffert (Eds.) (1983) J. B. Lippincott, Philadelphia.

2

The Paediatric Consultation

G. C. BENNET

It is hardly surprising that little consideration is given to the consultation in adult practice. Most adult patients present with a complaint, relate its characterisitics and effects to the surgeon who usually then proceeds to elicit a few further points in the history, particularly with regard to the functional effects of the disorder, examines the patient and comes to a provisional diagnosis. A relatively straightforward process. If the same technique is applied in paediatric practice it may not meet with the same degree of success. The doctor will fail to appreciate many unspoken pointers and clues and, as a result, will have more unsatisfactory consultations than need be the case. Such a consultation will undoubtedly adversely affect the parents opinion of the doctor's abilities which in turn will make the communication of explanations more difficult and the explanations themselves less credible.

Orthopaedic surgery has been described as the 'last bastion of the macho male'. Whilst a little unfair it does suggest that psychological subtlety is not foremost in the character of everyone in the speciality. Fortunately, however, although some sensitivity is required in conducting a paediatric consultation, a few simple guidelines can be used to make the process much simpler and more predictably successful. Although every child and family is obviously different and therefore so too is every consultation, there are certain common themes which, if applied, make the acquisition of interviewing and examining skills easier. Although surgeons vary in their approach it is worthwhile setting out a few of the ground rules used, often instinctively, by those practising predominantly in the paediatric field. It would be illogical to consider only one side of the consultation equation, namely the child and its family, so we will first look at the doctor and his clinic or consulting rooms.

Clinic organization

Whilst an appropriate physical setting is something that is taken for granted in a children's hospital, it may be more difficult to obtain in an adult environment. The waiting area should be reasonably spacious and comfortable with a variety of toys available. Sympathetic reception staff attuned to the inevitable noise and mess are invaluable. Childsized furniture is desirable both in the waiting area and in the consulting room itself where a few toys and books are useful as is enough space to see the child walk around. If this is not possible a corridor outside can be used for the same purpose.

An appointment system is essential. Whilst we all resent being kept waiting and become irritable as a result, trying to keep a handicapped or indeed a normal child amused in a waiting room for a couple of hours can become intolerable. The inevitable result will be a fractious child and a bad tempered parent, hardly the attitudes conducive to a friendly consultation. Whilst it is perfectly possible to examine an angry adult, it may be impossible to do so to a similarly disposed child.

Finally, there is a great deal to be said in favour of organizing specialized clinics for specific chronic disorders such as myelomeningocele or muscular dystrophy. By seeing several specialists and their supporting staff on the same day, multiple visits are avoided and all the necessary departments can gear their work load accordingly. An additional advantage for the parents is that it allows the exchange of experiences with others who have doubtless met with, and perhaps overcome, the same difficulties and this in itself may be therapeutic.

The doctor

The specific needs of a paediatric clinic are emphasized by the fact that the doctor may even dress differently! Some consider that a white coat frightens children. Whilst it is difficult to know whether it is the coat rather than the occupant that does so, there is something to be said for not wearing one. The price paid for this, however, is that by the end of the day there will be a variety of stains on one's trousers of which plaster of Paris is likely to be the least offensive. For perhaps the same reasons, many paediatricians seem to prefer bow ties!

A conscious attempt should be made to keep the consultation informal. Placing oneself on the opposite side of a desk from the patient is not the best start. If a desk must be used it is better to sit at the side. By definition, any consultation is a two way process. A child is unable to adapt its behaviour to differing circumstances so that, to help satisfactory communications by putting both the children and parents at their ease, a doctor must be prepared to modify his. There is little point in trying to be too dignified. Children are no respectors of person and their antics are likely to deflate pomposity, so it is better to be prepared to laugh at yourself or others will do so.

Just as all illness is not psychological so too is not all illness physical. One should try to place a particular illness within the context of the family. By creating the right atmosphere this may be possible. If the surgeon appears unsympathetic or uninterested then the family will not reward him with their confidences and any such underlying problems will remain undiscovered.

After introducing yourself make a point of using names, but first find out what the child is usually called as this often bears little resemblance to the name on the notes.

Whilst a counsel of perfection, Apley and McKeith's (1968) attitude that it is their fault if a child cries in their clinic makes a valid point.

The consultation

The aim of a consultation is to find out who thinks something is wrong, why they think something is wrong and then to discover what, if anything, is wrong. What we have already considered has been aimed at the creation of an atmosphere conducive to an exchange of information whereby these questions can be answered. Whereas in adult practice there is usually little difficulty in appreciating the purpose of a consultation, in a paediatric setting this may be much less straightforward. The whole process is simplified if one can discover at the outset who is making the complaint and why. The patient has obviously been brought to medical attention because he does not conform to someone's preconceived ideas of how a child should be at a particular age. Knowing who that person is and their knowledge of children makes evaluation of the complaint easier. For example a mother of five has plenty of experience in observing the normal in her own children and can readily appreciate any deviation from it. If she thinks something is wrong she is probably right. One can not expect the same astute observation from a mother of one. On entering the consulting room be on the look-out for any clues which may help resolve these questions. First and most obvious, who is present? Whilst there are obvious cultural differences, in the UK the child is usually brought to the clinic by its mother, sometimes accompanied by its siblings and this can be taken as the norm. Perhaps the most usual departure from this is a young first born child. Often then the father too will be present, usually carrying the vast amount of equipment that seems to accompany first born babies wherever they go. With this exception, the presence of a father, often as a silent observer, might mean that he is behind the complaint. Alternatively, and particularly in the case of the older child it may indicate joint parental ambition for their offspring, usually in a field of sporting endeavour such as gymnastics. A grandmother in the background, or more ominously, in the foreground taking over the role of protector of a baby from the natural mother may lead to problems. This is most often found in relation to a young, inexperienced and perhaps unmarried mother. The grandmother then is usually found to be behind the complaint. Such grandmothers may be trying to continue to exercise their hold over their own children by attempting to break their often fragile belief in their ability to take care of their child. Under such circumstances one should aim to boost their flagging confidence, perhaps at the expense of Granny. Particularly in the case of chronic handicap, the child and its mother may be accompanied by a physiotherapist or other health professional. Their views are worth listening to as they will certainly know the child better than you do and will have seen it perform in more natural and familiar surroundings. Often though, their presence will indicate that they wish to impress upon you the desirability of a particular course of treatment or the provision of a certain device or orthosis. On the other hand, they may be there to stop you suggesting an alternative (usually surgical) method of management. Be diplomatic! Whilst obviously generalizations, these observations often prove to be correct. It is fascinating to look out for such features and their discovery will brighten even the most mundane consultation. Certainly, anyone working in the field of paediatric orthopaedics, will have numerous examples of their own.

Why the complaint has been made is the next problem. A knowledge of disease in the community may prove to be useful. It is well known that when an osteosarcoma is diagnosed it is not uncommon to find other children from the same school or locality presenting with fairly vague limb complaints or ill-defined swellings. They all wish to be reassured that their usually innocuous lumps (often normal anatomical landmarks) are not malignant. It is very easy to miss the point of such a consultation. Alternatively parents bring their children up with minor complaints as they fear that, if not treated early, the child will grow up with a permanent deformity blaming them for their neglect. Such complaints may be unfairly dismissed as trivial.

The referral letter from the family doctor may be helpful in this respect. It might be full of otherwise unobtainable information on the family circumstances and background. On the other hand it may not! It at least offers a point at which to open the consultation: 'Dr McTavish says that Hamish has been limping for two months. Perhaps you could tell me about it.' Do not forget that the patient has been referred for a particular reason. Try to solve the problem posed. The doctor may have sent the child because he does not know what is wrong, because his reassurances and explanations have not been accepted, because the parents have insisted upon a specialist opinion or because investigations he could not undertake are required. Alternatively it may have been referred as a second specialist opinion. In this case tread carefully. Never give any hint of criticism of a colleague as there may be many reasons, of which you are unaware, for his having chosen certain courses of action even if the final result has turned out badly. Do not forget too that he is probably seeing your failures!

In the case of a young child address the first questions to its mother. Her observations are likely to be the most valuable and, whilst she may not always relate them in the clearest or most succinct manner, it is advisable to at least let her have her say. Not to give her this opportunity may lead to ill-feeling and a reluctance to accept advice proffered at the end of the consultation.

The child meantime can have a look at you. Whether he is ostensibly playing with toys, running around or sitting quietly he will undoubtedly be keeping an eye on you and his mother. By all means say hello but there is usually little point in asking even the most innocuous questions at this stage as they are likely to be met with a sullen silence which, once started, may continue throughout the consultation. He is waiting for a lead from his mother. Once he sees that you and she are friendly enough and that she trusts you, he is likely to adopt her attitude and later cooperation is very much more likely. You can meantime be assessing him. Although no child will behave naturally during a clinic visit, one can certainly learn something from their general demeanour. Most, however, either relapse into complete silence or, to the great embarrassment of their parents, run wild.

Although in the case of an older child or adolescent the history can be obtained directly from the patient, this may paradoxically complicate rather than simplify matters. Often the parents will interupt the child's story, perhaps because they feel they are taking too long 'the doctor's a busy man', because they are being inaccurate 'tell the doctor what you told me outside' or even in an attempt to put their child or themselves in a better light. Whilst it is difficult to stop them doing so, keep plugging away at the child for the rest of his story. This may not be easy, particularly in the case of adolescents who may be in open disagreement with their parents.

Hopefully by the end of all this a clear picture will have emerged as to what the problem is, what functional effect it is having and who is worried about it. At this stage go back to the beginning (pregnancy not conception) and build up a picture of the child's development. The detail required will depend upon the complaint. In congenital dislocation of the hip for example it would be worthwhile enquiring after breech position and amniocentesis and the results of neonatal hip testing would obviously be sought. In cerebral palsy problems during pregnancy, the method of delivery, whether resuscitation was required and whether the child was in a special care unit are all of direct relevance. So too with regard to motor milestones. Whilst little detail is required in the child who presents with intoeing due to femoral torsion, much more will be necessary if developmental delay is suspected. An outline of the milestones in motor development is shown in Table 2.1.

The family history of a disorder should not be ignored although often for differing reasons. In simple conditions such as flat feet, toe deformities or intoeing, the family experience of a disease may have a bearing on why they have brought the child to an orthopaedic clinic in the first place. If, in their childhood, a parent

Table 2.1. Motor milestones

6 weeks	Starts smiling
	Develops some head control
	Eyes fixate on objects
4 months	Reaches for objects
6 months	Sits for short time without support
	Bears full weight if held erect
	Transfers objects from one hand to the other
9 months	Can pull to standing position
	Stands holding onto furniture
10 months	Sits very steadily. Can right itself if pushed off balance
11 months	Walks holding onto furniture
13 months	Independent walking with broad based gait
	Uses pinch grip
18 months	Goes up and down stairs

NB   All these times are approximations and there is a wide variation of normality. The sequence, however, is the same in all children.

had to wear splints for knock knees or had shoe alterations for intoeing, they may, not unreasonably, expect the same treatment for their offspring. Similarly, if a grandmother has a bad hip they may be worried that the child has the same disorder. Once such information is available explanations can be aimed at specific points and appropriate reassurance given. In more serious conditions such as muscular dystrophy the family history is obviously of great relevance and may be vital so as to allow the appropriate genetic counselling to be given. Even in the most unlikely circumstances knowledge of the family may be useful. Not infrequently, the supposedly clumsy child merely has the misfortune to follow an exceptionally athletic older sibling.

Examination

Height and weight can be recorded on arrival by the clinic nurse and the data entered upon the appropriate growth chart. Before attempting to formally examine the patient have a chat with them. Ask them to show you their toy or remark on

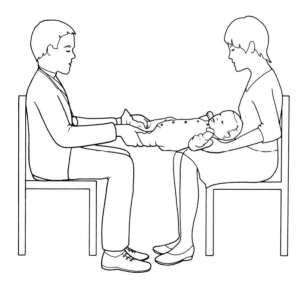

Fig. 2.1 Examination of a young child

some obviously new item of clothing that they are wearing. They will probably be proud of them and will be gratified by your interest as all children like being the centre of attention. It is always worthwhile asking their permission to examine them. Once such permission is given there is seldom any problem. Next decide where the examination will take place. With young children their cooperation may depend upon their maintaining contact with their mother. Accept this and proceed with the examination on their mother's knee. (Fig. 2.1).

In the case of the older child, before undressing starts, get them to walk around and assess their gait. Ask them to walk on tiptoe and on their heels and have them perform a Gower's test. At this stage ask them to to take off some of their clothes, usually socks, shoes and trousers in the case of their hips. Although having them undress at this stage rather than earlier takes a little longer, it is worth the delay. Apart from the fact that it is undesirable to have patients sitting with their clothes off, some children associate the act of undressing with being kept in hospital, thus explaining the reluctance that is sometimes found at this stage. Once the part in question has been examined remove the rest of their clothes, with the exception of their underwear, so that a general examination can be made. Older children should be offered privacy. Uncovering and examining only the part about which the complaint is made lacks conviction. Quite apart from the fact that unexpected pathology may be found elsewhere, the examiniation is not only concerned with diagnosis. Having obviously performed a thorough examination will add to the authority of later explanations which, as a consequence, will be more easily accepted. If it is anticipated that any part of the examination will cause discomfort or distress, that part should be left until last.

Specific examination of the hip follows along routine lines. Testing for hip stability in the neonate is dealt with in Chapter 4. Gait is examined. What, if any, abnormality is present? Is there a limp, if so which side? Perform a Trendelenberg test remembering that in some children, for example with hip subluxation or Perthes disease, a positive result may be delayed. Check the leg lengths. In older children this may easily be performed in the standard manner with a tape measure, whereas, in younger children or babies lack of cooperation may make this impossible. Under these circumstances the alternative method outlined in Fig. 2.2 is useful. Check for wasting of the thighs or buttocks. The latter can easily be appreciated by having the child lie prone and asking him to tighten his bottom and palpating each buttock, when any significant difference is very evident. At the same time the back can be examined for stigmata of spinal dysraphism.

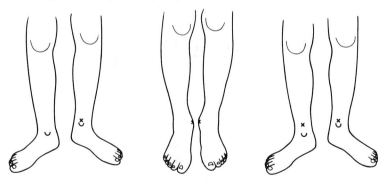

Fig. 2.2 Leg length measurement. Mark the medial malleolus of the shorter leg with an ink pen or felt-tip. With the pelvis level and the legs extended, press the marked malleolus against the medial side of the opposite lower leg. This leaves the imprint of the cross on the longer leg. The difference in leg length, that is X to the medial malleolus, is then easily measured.

Hip movements should be measured in the prone and supine positions. Abnormalities of tone will be noted at this stage.

The torsional profile (Staheli 1977) is outlined in Fig. 2.3. Once hip examination is completed the rest of the lower limbs should be examined as, particularly in the case of a limp, the cause may well lie somewhere other than the hip. If it seems indicated, a full neurological examination of the lower limbs should be performed.

Once all this has been done the diagnosis may be clear, suspected or obscure.

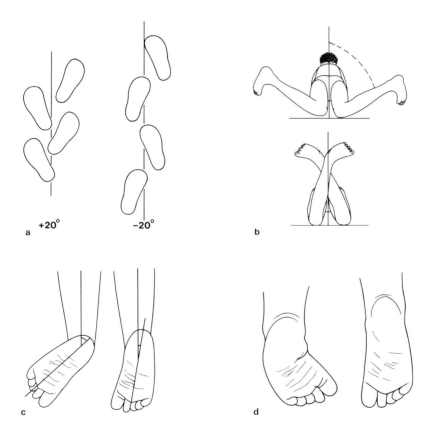

Fig. 2.3 The torsional profile.

(a) The foot progression angle. Have the child walk around a little until they stop feeling self-conscious. Then estimate the angle the foot makes with the line of progression. A positive value denotes out-toeing and a negative intoeing. The rest of the examination is performed with the child prone.

(b) Hip rotation. Used as an indication of femoral torsion. Internal and external rotation is measured and recorded.

(c) The thigh foot angle. Flex the knee to 90° and with light pressure, place the foot in the neutral position. Look down on the plantar surface of the foot and estimate the angle the axis of the foot makes with the line of the thigh. This is taken as a measure of tibial torsion. A positive value denotes external torsion and a negative internal.

(d) Foot shape. If metatarsus adductus is contributing to a gait abnormality its presence is readily appreciated at this stage of the examination.

Radiographs may be indicated either to help elucidate the diagnosis or to support any subsequent reassurance that no significant pathology is present.

If the diagnosis is clear and no treatment is required, explanations are in order. The phrase to avoid at this point is 'there is nothing wrong'. Obviously someone thinks there is or the parents would not have gone to the trouble of coming to see you. Explanations should be given in a way that the parents can reasonably be expected to understand. Doctors tend to take their ability to do this for granted and any failure of comprehension is presumed to be the fault of the parents. This is often a mistaken assumption. Use diagrams and drawings to explain and if necessary give them explanatory handouts which can be prepared for the more common complaints such as intoeing. If they do not appear to understand go through it again or ask them to repeat what you have said. This is particularly useful in the case of those parents whose English may be poor and it also serves as a feedback against which you can check the effectiveness of your explanations. All this may help you avoid that most embarrassing of situations, namely overhearing the parents asking the nurse 'what did he say?'.

Even if the diagnosis is not clearcut a plan of management can still be decided upon. This does not necessarily mean launching into a series of evermore complicated investigations. If you have excluded serious disease explain this and, if necessary, arrange to see the child again with the proviso that, should the problem become more severe before the next appointment, you would be happy to see them sooner. If further investigations do seem necessary, explain why. If admission is required offer to let them see round the ward or arrange for them to attend a preadmission programme if one exists. If at all possible, particularly in the case of younger children, offer the parents the option of being resident. Something good can be said about (almost) all children so, at the end of the consultation, try to find something nice to say. It will give a boost to the parents and make them feel better about the whole consultation. Indeed such a remark is often remembered and repeated for a surprisingly long time. Additionally, it will do your reputation no harm: 'what a nice man'.

References and recommended reading

Apley J. & McKeith R. (1968) *The Child and His Symptoms*. Blackwell Scientific Publications, Oxford.
Rang M. (1982) *The Easter Seal Guide to Childrens Orthopaedics*. The Easter Seal Society, Ontario.
Staheli L. (1977) Torsional deformities. *Paediatric Clinics of North America*, **24**, 799–811.
Stone F. (1984) Interviewing children and parents. In *Children; a Handbook for Children's Doctors*. Gray P. & Cockburn F. pp. 45–9. Pitman Publishing, London.

3

Congenital Abnormalities of the Femur

I. P. TORODE

Introduction

In an attempt to cover the information relating to the diversity of conditions which might fall under the all encompassing title of 'congenital abnormalities of the femur', one must first define the limits of the discussion. Merely to list all the possible conditions reported in the textbooks on congenital abnormalities is of little benefit.

Four conditions are presented in this chapter together with their principles of management in the hope that the reader will then be equipped to use these principles in other situations in which patients have femoral deficiencies whether the aetiology be congenital, vascular, neoplastic or traumatic.

The conditions are:

1 congenital hemihypertrophy/hemiatrophy;
2 congenital coxa vara;
3 congenital short femur;
4 proximal femoral focal deficiency.

It is recognized that other texts have presented different classifications, but no matter what terms are applied to the individual conditions, their presenting problem remains the same and their treatment requirements should be tailored to the needs of each condition, rather than to their artificial title.

In this chapter and its accompanying illustrations, the reader will immediately be reminded of the deformities due to dysplasias, for example Ollier disease (Fig. 3.1) where the deformity is not that dissimilar to congenital short femur with deficiencies in length as well as angulation, or that of fibrous dysplasia with the shepherd's crook deformity where the incompetent bone will not support the weight of the body without realignment of the proximal femur into valgus.

Whilst it is beyond the scope of this chapter to give a detailed discussion on the inheritance pattern of congenital disease, they essentially come under three categories:

1 Mendelian disorders, where there is a single gene defect which regularly gives predictable patterns of inheritance;

2   chromosomal disorders, where there is involvement of a sufficient number of genes to give visual changes on the microscopic examination of the chromosomes;
3   multifactorial, where there is a combination of genetic and environmental factors.

It has been estimated that 90% of congenital malformations are genetically influenced, 60% being multifactorial, 20% Mendelian disorders, 10% due to chromosomal disorders and 10% due to maternal viral infections, for example rubella (Cowell 1978). Of the topics under discussion, only congenital coxa vara appears to have a reasonably predictable inheritance pattern and the aetiology of the other groups remains a mystery (Fig. 3.2). Typical examples have been noted as being due to environmental agents, for example proximal femoral focal deficiency as seen caused by thalidomide, when ingested by the mother in the first trimester of pregnancy.

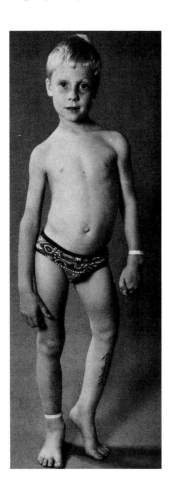

Fig. 3.1 Boy with Ollier disease resulting in a short and angulated femur mimicking, but not truly, a congenital deformity.

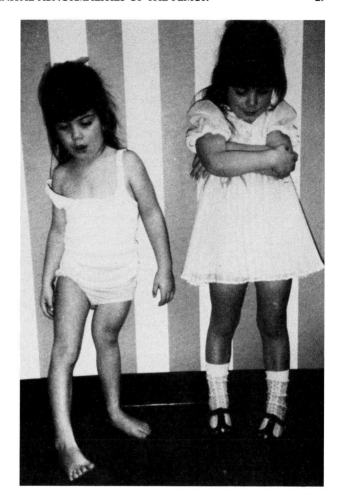

Fig. 3.2 Twin girls identical in all respects save that one has a congenital short femur affecting her left leg.

1. Congenital hemihypertrophy/hemiatrophy

Congenital hypertrophy rather than congenital hemiatrophy appears to have become the accepted term for the situation where an infant is born with one half of its body a different size to the other half. The extremities are normal in appearance, except for differences in length and girth and in the complete form of the condition, the difference in size extends to include the trunk and head and there may even be differences in size of the eyes and the texture of hair, nails and skin (Bryan *et al.* 1958).

Hemiatrophy is thus thought to be the appropriate term for situations where there is a deficiency in supply, particularly neural, whereas hemihypertrophy is used in those situations where there is an excessive supply, either lymphatic or vascular, with secondary overgrowth of other tissues. The term congenital is used somewhat loosely in this context in that the abnormality is often overlooked at birth, except in the more severe varieties and is usually recognized later on as a leg length discrepancy. Many cases of hypertrophy are partial or segmental in that only one limb, usually the lower limb, and part of the trunk, is involved. The syndrome was first described by Wagner in 1839 and there are a number of classifications including that of Ward and Lerner (1947) which served to illustrate the differences between the idiopathic group and those for which a cause can be found. Careful examination of these children is required to rule out these secondary and acquired causes of asymmetry including neurofibromatosis, hyperpituitarism, A-V malformations, Milroy disease, elephantiasis, Wilms tumour and others.

Furthermore, there are syndromes described that include asymmetry of growth, for example Silver syndrome (Tachdjian 1982), Klippel–Trenaunay syndrome and Proteus syndrome (Temtamy & Rogers 1976) (Fig. 3.3). The hypertrophy in these syndromes, however, approaches that of gigantism, rather than the problems of femoral asymmetry that are to be discussed under this heading.

The inheritance of congenital hemihypertrophy has not been clearly defined, although familial cases have been described (Scott 1935). In other series mental deficiency has been noted in up to 20% of cases (Morris & MacGillivray 1955). Associated anomalies, for example syndactylism and polydactylism, have been found in approximately 50% of cases (Bryan *et al.* 1958).

The clinical problem of hemihypertrophy is basically one of leg length, and occasionally foot size, discrepancy. Shoe modifications and/or slipper inserts will adequately compensate for the difference in shoe sizes.

Measurement of limb length

The methods of estimating limb length discrepancy include clinical measurements, utilizing a tape measure and standing blocks and radiological measurements including teleroentgenograms, orthoroentgenograms and scanograms and the CT scanning method.

Tape measure

Although the use of the tape measure may appear at first too basic to consider mentioning, it will provide the true and apparent leg lengths and sequential lengths. It provides an easy, inexpensive and readily repeatable check on measurements obtained by more technically advanced methods.

Blocks

The use of standing blocks of graduated increments gives the examiner the most accurate guide to the amount that needs to be added to the patient's limb to level the pelvis. Not only is this an inexpensive and reproduceable method, but also takes into account deficiencies in heel size and pelvic asymmetry which are omitted if only the femur and tibia are measured. The use of standing blocks also gives the patient some idea of the effect that lengthening one limb may have on their body position.

Radiological methods

Teleroentgenogram

This technique utilizes a single, long radiographic film, usually exposed at a tube to film distance of 72 inches, to show the entire length of both extremities at once.

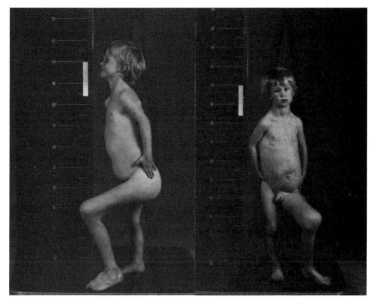

Fig. 3.3 A young boy with Proteus sydrome whose left leg approximates adults size even though his chronological age is approximately 5 years.

There are some inherent inaccuracies in this technique due to magnification of the image caused by the divergence of the X-ray beams (Green *et al.* 1946). The single film is most useful in younger patients with shorter limbs and where angular deformities need to be measured and recorded.

Scanogram

This is a modification of the orthoroentgenogram described by Bell and Thompson (1950). The procedure is useful for older patients and combines the accuracy of the orthoroentgenogram with the convenience of a smaller film as the film is moved beneath the patient for successive exposures of the desired parts of the limb. The technique also incorporates the use of a radio-opaque ruler so that measurement can be taken directly off the X-ray film (Fig. 3.4).

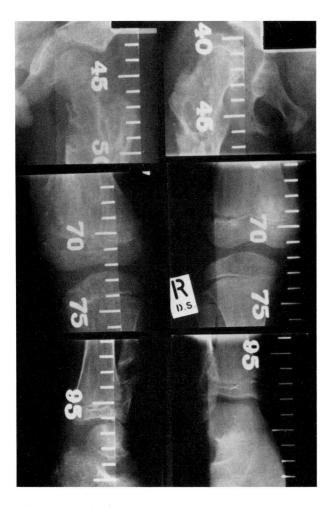

Fig. 3.4 A scanogram which incorporates the use of radio-opaque rule to obtain direct measurements without the problems of magnification.

CT scan method

This technique utilizing the vast advances made in radiographic imaging, provides limb length measurements from the scout film obtained on the regular CT scanner. The patient lies on the scanning platform, the scout film is obtained and a cursor is placed over bony landmarks at desired intervals and the distance between these cursor points is generated by the computer of the CT scanner (Helms 1984) (Fig. 3.5).

The computer data generated are expressed in terms that far exceed the accuracy demanded by our surgical techniques, but nonetheless do provide an accurate method of limb length measurement and the data are stored conveniently and can be regenerated at any time. The X-rays or hard copy produced by the CT scan are also in a form much smaller and more conveniently stored than that of, for example, an orthoroentgenogram. Where the foot is a significant component of the limb length discrepancy a foot plate can be used as the lowest cursor point on each limb.

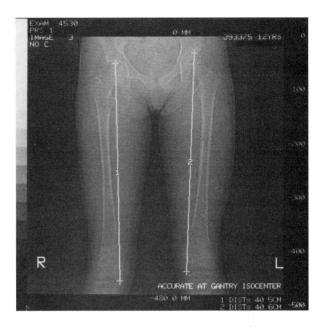

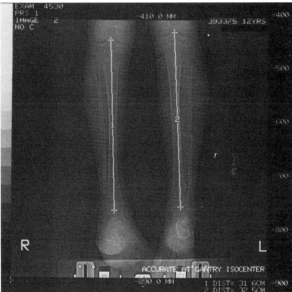

Fig. 3.5 This illustrates the technique utilizing a CT scanner to measure limb length. The cursor can be placed at any two points on the screen and the distance between those two points measured accurately.

Growth of limbs

The problem of patients with idiopathic congenital hemihypertrophy is that of a limb length discrepancy of a degree that can be managed either by an epiphysiodesis, or by a limb shortening procedure. In the growing child there are three commonly used techniques for estimating growth of the limb:

1   growth remaining method (Green & Anderson);
2   rule of thumb technique (Menelaus);
3   straight line graph (Moseley).

Growth remaining method

The data relating to leg length in children from the study by Anderson and Green was initially published in 1948 and subsequently follow-up data was published in 1963. From this data growth curves have been produced and graphs illustrating the growth remaining in the distal femur and proximal tibia have been formulated. Utilizing these graphs, the growth remaining in a particular growth centre at a particular age can be estimated and from this information the desired time for an epiphysiodesis can be estimated (Green & Anderson 1946, 1955, 1960). Obviously the accuracy of this technique will improve by incorporating as many points as possible on these curves and any deviations from the standard curve can be recognized.

The Menelaus technique

Menelaus (1966) published a technique for estimating the timing of an epiphyseal arrest, which has been derived from the rate of growth of part of the Anderson–Green curve that is applicable to the timing of epiphyseal arrest, i.e. from the age of 10 years to maturity. White and Stubbings (1944) and Menelaus (1966) have suggested the femoral epiphysis grows at 3/8 inch per year and the proximal tibial epiphysis at 1/4 inch per year. During this period and utilizing this knowledge and repeated measurements of the limb length discrepancy will reveal the annual increase/decrease of this discrepancy, the expected discrepancy at maturity (Greulich & Pyle 1959) will be known and thus the age at which an epiphyseal arrest would need to be performed to make up this discrepancy can be calculated.

Moseley straight line method (Mosely 1977)

By an imaginative and ingenious method of data manipulation, Moseley has prepared a method on the basis of the straight line graph for recording leg length discrepancies and preparing predictions of discrepancies at maturity. This method was published in 1977 and on a single page graph, allows one to plot the measurement of both legs and the skeletal age of the child and, by utilizing the reference slopes, also contained on the page, the effect of the appropriate epiphyiodesis can be predicted. As with the previous methods, the more measurements that are plotted on the graph, the greater will be the accuracy of prediction. It should be borne in mind that the data to provide the above methods came from studies now almost 40 years old.

Surgery in congenital hemihypertrophy where indicated, will be either an epiphysiodesis in the distal femur, proximal tibia, or both, or limb shortening of either femur or tibia. Although a number of techniques of epiphysiodesis have been presented, the methods are essentially those which remove or destroy an epiphysis and those which employ a device to prevent longitudinal growth (Goff 1960).

The epiphyseal destructive methods largely revolve around that procedure described by Phemister (1933) or the varying modifications thereof (Ward & Lerner 1947, Blount & Clark 1949). Other methods using cryoprobes or percutaneous drilling (Canale *et al.* 1986, Ogilvie 1986) have yet to become universally popular, although in the future, particularly with improved imaging, these techniques may become the method of choice.

The most common method of mechanically preventing epiphyseal growth is by using staples (Blount & Clark 1949). The theoretical advantages of having a safety valve by continued growth after removal of the staples should the procedure have been performed prematurely, seems to be outweighed by the lack of predictability of their effect and the apparent delay in the onset of their effect in slowing growth. Nonetheless the epiphyseal stapling remains an effective method of correction of angular deformity in growing children.

Shortening

There are many different ways of shortening a limb and the methods described date back to the middle of last century (Rissoli as quoted by Goff 1960). In the femur the three most commonly used methods are:

1 subtrochanteric resection with fixation by a nail-plate device;
2 open femoral resection with intramedullary nail fixation;
3 closed femoral shortening and intramedullary fixation, utilizing instruments specifically designed for that purpose as described by Winquist *et al.* (1978).

Each of these methods has its own particular advocates and, although the third method has some advantages, it is technically difficult and is not possible without the specialized instruments.

In certain circumstances, tibial shortening provides a simple method for correcting limb length. By step-cut resection and interfragmentary screw fixation, shortening up to approximately 3.5 cm can be obtained without undue morbidity and with rapid union.

Although epiphysiodesis has proved a reliable method of equalizing limb length in the growing child with a discrepancy from 1.5 to 5 cm, there will be situations where the discrepancy will be greater than 2 cm, but the growth remaining is inadequate to allow for an epiphysiodesis or where the situation is changing close to maturity such that the final discrepancy can not be reliably estimated. Under these circumstances, a tibial resection of up to 3.5 cm or femoral resection of up to 6 cm can achieve equally satisfying results.

In summary, the problems of a patient with congenital hemihypertrophy are primarily those of a leg length inequality and can be managed by an appropriate epiphysiodesis, or in certain circumstances, a femoral or tibial shortening.

2. Congenital coxa vara

The term congenital coxa vara was presented by Hofmeister in 1894 (Babb *et al.* 1949) with the deformity first being described by Fiorani in 1881 (Zadek 1935) and, although there may be some doubt as to the accuracy of the diagnosis from those times, congenital coxa vara remains an entity in its own right. At first glance the deformity may be thought to be part of the spectrum of congenital short femur but there are several features unique to these patients which justify its being considered separately.

Congenital coxa vara must be distinguished from that arising secondary to other causes. These conditions can include Morquio's osteochondrodystrophy, cleidocranial dysostosis, metaphyseal dysostosis, multiple epiphyseal dysplasia, achondroplasia and epiphyseal injury due to trauma or infection.

It has been suggested that the term congenital coxa vara is a misnomer as the deformity is not usually recognized until the child presents with a limp in the unilateral deformity or a waddling gait with a bilateral deformity (Hensinger & Jones 1981). However, the deformity has been reported at the age of 18 months and in hindsight many of the children who are subsequently diagnosed probably had signs recognizable at an earlier age (Almond 1956, Fisher & Waskowitz 1972). Infantile coxa vara may be a more appropriate term.

The patients are typically of short stature, often with hyperlordosis of the lumbar spine, particularly in bilateral cases. The affected hip is seen to have a decreased range of abduction and internal rotation. The greater trochanter is prominent and a positive Trendelenberg sign is present. Signs of a congenital dislocation of the hip are of course absent. There is also a leg length discrepancy which appears to be slightly in excess of that due to the varus deformity of the neck alone. Radiographically the femoral neck is in varus with the proximal femoral epiphyseal plate being more vertical than normal. Although radiographs taken on presentation may not show the typical triangular fragment on the medial aspect of the femoral neck adjacent to the epiphyseal plate, it has been demonstrated (Pauwels 1976) that this radiographic feature can usually be found by appropriate rotation of the limb bringing the 'pseudoarthrosis' into the plane of the X-ray beam (Fig. 3.6). The neck shaft angle in the newborn would be expected to be approximately 150° but in congenital coxa vara, the angle is 120° or less.

The reason for this deformity remains unclear. While Alsberg (1899) suggested increased intrauterine pressure as an aetiology and Nilsonne (1928) felt the cause to be an embryonic vascular disorder, Hoffa (1905) recognized that the deformity resulted from a disturbance of the epiphysis. There are, however, two distinct possibilities and each may well contribute to the deformity. The first possibility is that there is a biological insufficiency of the proximal epiphyseal plate which, in the infant, involves not only the femoral head, but also the superior margin of the femoral neck and the greater trochanter. If there is an insufficiency of the enchondral ossification of the superior margin of the femoral neck, then the maturation of that part of the femur will be slowed, leading to a delay in completion of the ossification of the femoral neck and a varus attitude of the proximal femoral epiphyseal plate. The second contributing factor is based on mechanical grounds where it is postulated that the femoral neck, being composed of mechanically insufficient cartilage, is unable to withstand the stresses of weightbearing thereby aggravating the varus deformity (Pauwels 1976) and preventing remodelling into a valgus attitude. Furthermore, the defect on the lateral aspect of the triangular fragment is a deficiency in the bone due to the stresses applied thus a stress fracture is created which fails to heal because of the continuing malalignment of forces.

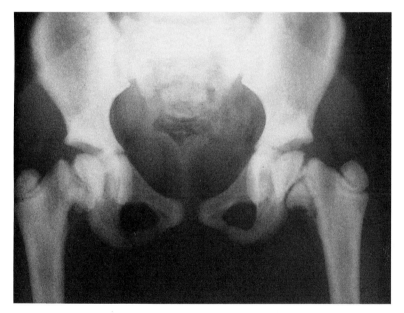

Fig. 3.6 Radiograph demonstrating bilateral congenital coxa vara with the metaphyseal defect and the triangular metaphyseal fragment between the 'defect' and the growth plate.

Thus there are several features distinguishing congenital coxa vara from the coxa vara seen in the congenital short femur. The first of these is that the varus is due to deformity in the most proximal portion of the femur, the severity of which is a function of the verticality of the epiphyseal plate. The deformity is progressive unless corrected surgically. If the plate is not corrected adequately and shear stress across the plate remains, then the deformity will recur. This is in distinction to the coxa vara of the congenital short femur, the varus deformity of which is static and is due to a more distal deformity rather than one in the most proximal epiphyseal region. Another feature of distinction is the inheritance pattern which would appear to be autosomal dominant with incomplete penetrance as evidenced by the increased frequency of congenital coxa vara in communities which have remained geographically, and thus genetically separate (Almond 1956, Blount 1949, Fisher 1972, Marchetti & Faldini 1968, Binazzi 1986).

With regard to treatment, there are two areas to approach, the first obviously being correction of the varus attitude of the femoral neck and the second the leg length discrepancy. The principles of management of limb length discrepancy have been covered in the previous section and will not be discussed further.

Correction of the varus deformity can only be by surgery and the relevant decisions are those of timing and method. Delaying surgery too long may result in severe deformity, but premature surgery may result in recurrence.

With respect to timing, a study by Weinstein et al. (1984) suggested that the angle of the ephiphyseal plate is the key determinant. They have proposed that a Helgrenrener Epiphyseal angle (HE) (Fig. 3.7) of 60° or more required correction, an HE angle of 45°–60°, observation and that one of less than 45° could be expected to correct spontaneously. This concept is not dissimilar to that of Pauwels (1976).

Although epiphysiodesis of the greater trochanter can result in correction of a

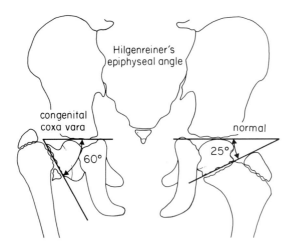

Fig. 3.7 Diagramatic representation of Helgrenreiner epiphyseal angle of 60° in congenital coxa vara as opposed to 25° in the normal.

varus deformity, the amount likely to be obtained is unpredictable. Thus a valgus osteotomy of the proximal femur is the most logical and reliable procedure. There are essentially three methods of correction of the deformity:

1   Osteotomy followed by hip spica. Although it is a simple task to perform an inter-trochanteric femoral osteotomy and to place a child in a hip spica, there is significant incidence of loss of correction in the postoperative period with recurrence of the deformity.

2   Osteotomy plus fixation:

a   A series of patients studied at the Rizzoli Institute revealed that an osteotomy using a screw-pin fixation achieved consistently good results. The screw-pins are left long and pass through the subcutaneous tissues and skin and are incorporated into the hip spica (Fig. 3.8) (Binazzi 1986, Marchetti & Faldini 1968.)

b   Tachdjian (1982) has illustrated a similar method involving an external fixator to maintain the correction.

c   Internal fixation by means of a small blade plate device to fix and hold the osteotomy in the corrected position with support from hip spica cast.

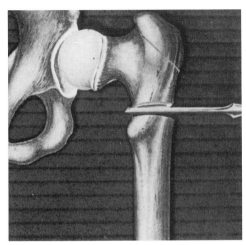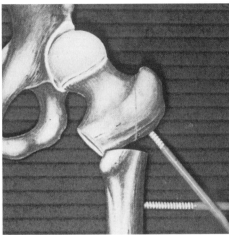

Fig. 3.8 Intertrochanteric osteotomy as described by Marchetti utilizing pins and plaster for fixation.

3   Osteotomy utilizing the stability obtained by bone realignment. The principle of this technique is the basis of the method described by Pauwels (1976). The correctly performed osteotomy provides intrinsic stability which is futher secured by wire fixation (Fig. 3.9).

Other techniques utilizing carpentry methods have been described by Amstutz and Wilson (1960) and Pyllkanen (1960).

Summary

Congenital coxa vara is a condition with a particular inheritance pattern and a particular bony deformity which probably results from a biologic insufficiency in the ossification of the proximal femur and is aggravated by the physiologic stresses applied across a mechanically insufficient weightbearing structure.

Congenital short femur and proximal femoral focal deficiency

These two groups are introduced together as they are frequently listed under the single diagnosis of proximal femoral focal deficiency. To pursue that approach, however, serves only to confuse the reader and fails to give direction to the surgeon in management and to indicate prognosis to the parents of the patient.

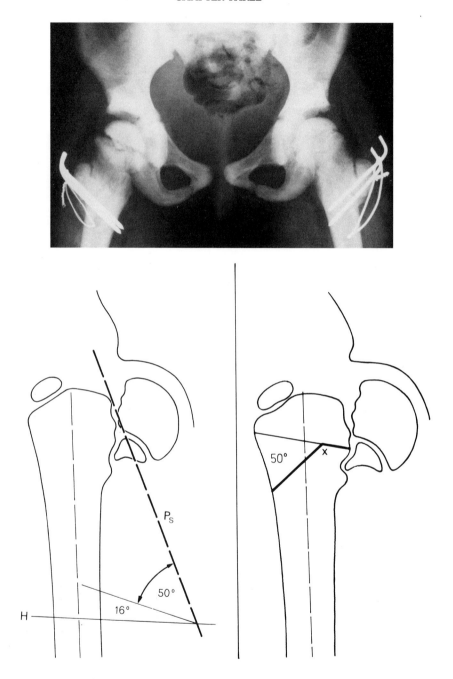

Fig. 3.9 Postoperative X-ray after Pauwels intertrochanteric osteotomy with tension band wiring.

The well known classifications of Aitken (1969) and Amstutz and Wilson (1962) have demonstrated that one can define various subgroups of femoral deficiency on radiographic appearances, but it must be borne in mind that these appearances change with the age of the patient and the eventual number of subgroups is defined only by the number of patients seen. This spectrum has clearly been documented by Hamanishi (1980).

On clinical grounds where the patients have growth deficiency of the femur greater than that of the modest leg length discrepancies as described under congenital coxa vara and congenital hemihypertrophy up to the most extreme femoral deficiency imaginable, they will be seen to fall into two main groups. These groups have been termed congenital short femur and proximal femoral focal deficiency.

In dealing with any congenital abnormality, one must recognize that the extremes of any sub-group may require a compromise of the treatment guidelines which have been outlined for the ideal case. For example, in dealing with a case of congenital short femur, an associated short distal segment and a severe foot anomaly that one might see with a fibular hemimelia, attempts to avoid amputation and the pursuit of leg length equality through surgery may prove a wasteful, painful and time-consuming expedition towards an end point which was obvious to the uninvolved observer at the outset (Fig. 3.10).

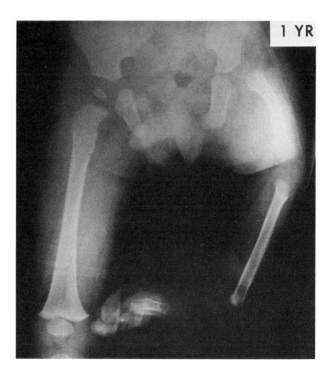

Fig. 3.10 Radiograph of boy at 1 year with a left congenital short femur in association with tibial hemimelia and associated foot deformity.

3. Congenital short femur

In this group, the deficiency of the femur, although marked, is less severe than that of the true proximal femoral focal deficiency (PFFD). In relation to the 'normal' side the foot is approximately at the midtibial level. In infancy the child lies with the leg in lateral rotation and abduction with the hip and knee flexed. The flexion deformities however are not severe and will decrease in severity over the first year of life. (Fig. 3.11).

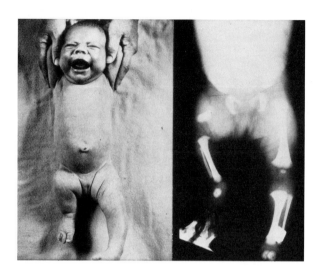

Fig. 3.11 Clinical photograph of an infant with the posture typical of both proximal focal deficiency and congenital short femur.

There will be cruciate insufficiency within the affected knee as described by Torode and Gillespie (1983) which will become more obvious as the child grows and the knee flexion contracture resolves. The valgus deformity of the knee, initially disguised by the chubbiness of the leg lying in lateral rotation and flexion will be much more evident (Fig. 3.12).

Radiographically, the initial picture may be unclear due to the posture. In a short space of time, however, the typical appearance of the short femur with a bulbous proximal end (Fixsen & Lloyd-Roberts 1974) is seen (Fig. 3.13). The proximal end of the ossified femur lies more proximal and lateral than normal which has led, in some cases, to its being misdiagnosed as congenital dislocation of the hip. Even though the proximal portion is in varus and retroversion, however, there is no defect in the radiolucent cartilagenous neck and trochanter, so that the term proximal femoral focal deficiency in this group is inappropriate.

By childhood years the proximal femur ossifies revealing a coxa vara which, in contradistinction to the congenital coxa vara described previously, is static and to the true proximal femoral focal deficiency where the progression of varus occurs through a fragile or defective cartilagenous bridge. The affected femur is 40–60% of the length of the normal side, with a lateral bow and sclerosis in the femoral shaft. The distal femur has a valgus deformity with hypoplasia of the femoral

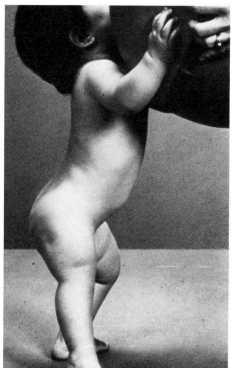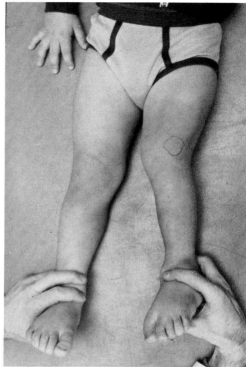

Fig. 3.12 Photographs showing that the contractures at the knee are not fixed and can be easily stretched out and with the knee in extension the gross valgus deformity is evident.

condyles, particularly the lateral condyle. Thus clinically, the picture of the child with a congenital short femur is that of a limb length discrepancy of approximately 20% with the limb lying in external rotation. On clinical examination, gross anteroposterior laxity is felt within the valgus knee joint (Fig. 3.14). Note that the cruciate laxity does not present as an unstable knee in day-to-day activities as one might expect knowing the extent of the deficiency within the knee articulation. Furthermore because the child stands with the leg in external rotation and the foot in extension, the valgus knee can be disguised. Nonetheless in spite of the marked deficiency the below knee segment is usually relatively normal and in this situation the aim of management in most instances will be leg length equalization.

Treatment

Nonsurgical

Options to maintain leg length equality include shoe lifts through to extension prostheses. As will be outlined, surgery is aimed at obtaining equality in length with both lengthening and epiphysiodesis. However, an aid of one sort or another will be needed until maturity has been attained and the end of the surgical programme reached (Fig. 3.15).

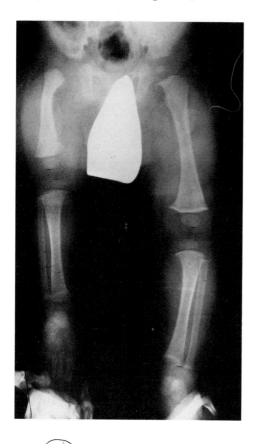

Fig. 3.13 Congenital short femur illustrating the varus femoral neck with sclerosis of the femoral shaft and hypoplastic femoral condyle. The valgus deformity is also evident.

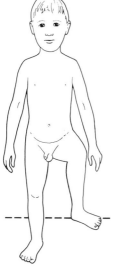

Leg length 20–30%

Valgus knee

A–P laxity knee

Flexion deformities
  not fixed

Foot midtibial level

Fig. 3.14 Clinical signs of congenital short femur.

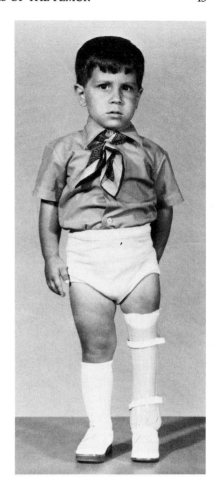

Fig. 3.15 Boy with congenital short femur needing to wear an extension prosthesis to equalize the left limb length.

Surgical

The surgical steps are outlined individually as it is the author's belief that lengthening a straight bone is a much less difficult task than lengthening an angulated or curved segment. Attempts to combine an often difficult lengthening procedure with either rotation or angular correction will jeopardize what may have been an otherwise successful undertaking.

Correction of *hip varus.* An osteotomy of the proximal femur utilizing a simple device such as K-wires or a small blade plate, supplemented by hip spica cast, has been universally successful in correcting the varus of the proximal femur. This not only improves the alignment, but usually gains approximately 2 cm in length, depending on the extent of the pre-existing varus deformity, the amount of correction obtained and the actual length of the femoral neck. At the time of correction of the hip varus, the external rotation deformity due to the retroversion of the femoral neck can also be corrected quite simply (Fig. 3.16).

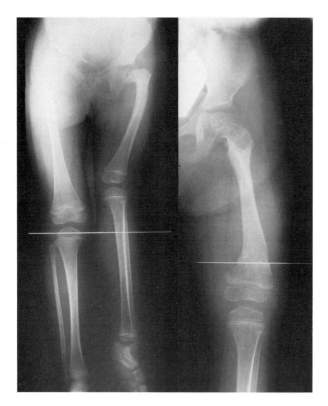

Fig. 3.16 Pre- and postoperative radiographs showing the pre-operative coxa vara, sclerosis of the shaft of the femur and valgus at the knee joint. Postoperative film shows correction of the hip varus and the knee valgus by abduction and adduction osteotomies respectively.

Correction of *knee valgus.* A transverse osteotomy of the distal femur utilizing a section of fibula as a graft to maintain an opening laterally based wedge will correct the knee valgus and also gain a significant amount of length. Once again, simple fixation, such as crossed wires and a plaster cast, will suffice to maintain the correction. Often, however, the fibular graft wedged into the opening osteotomy will be found to give adequate stability (Fig. 3.17).

Both these procedures as outlined serve not only to correct the alignment of the femur, but also to gain a few precious centimetres of length. The osteotomies should be performed before the age of 8 years, so that the discrepancy remaining can be calculated and the next steps planned. It appears that osteotomies at an early age can also stimulate growth of the bone and thus also provide a small gain in length in excess of that expected from the geometric correction of the malaligned limb.

Leg lengthening. Using the knowledge that the ratio of the femoral lengths of the affected limb to the unaffected limb at maturity will be approximately the same ratio as in infancy the predicted discrepancy can be estimated. The bonus in length obtained by the osteotomies described is subtracted from the estimated discrepancy, giving the deficit that needs to be made up by both epiphysiodesis and limb lengthening. A study of lengthening procedures performed in children with femoral deficiencies revealed that one should limit attempted gain to approximately 20% of the affected segment length (Gillespie & Torode 1983).

It is conceivable that the situation could arise where the amount required by femoral lengthening might be greatly in excess of that 20% estimated and thus one should consider the possibility that two limb lengthenings might be required. If one has already realigned the limb appropriately by the age of 8 to 10 years, then it is possible to perform two lengthening procedures, separated by several years that would allow full maturation of the grafted segment of the femur.

The actual technique of lengthening is not critical, although the author prefers that described by Wagner (1971), bearing in mind that the cruciate insufficiency of the knee predisposes to posterior subluxation of the tibia on the femur (Fig. 3.18). In an attempt to prevent this, the hamstrings, iliotibial band and biceps tendons should be lengthened prophylactically. Emphasis on knee motion during period of lengthening is often directed towards flexion but it should be remembered that subluxation of the tibia on the femur is always preceded by loss of extension of the knee joint. Dislocation of the hip has been seen by the author and subluxation has also been reported (Salai et al.1985).

While the author's experience with limb lengthening has largely evolved from the principles as outlined by Wagner (1971), the advent and increasing use of distraction epiphysiolysis must be recognized (Mezhenina et al. 1984). This method

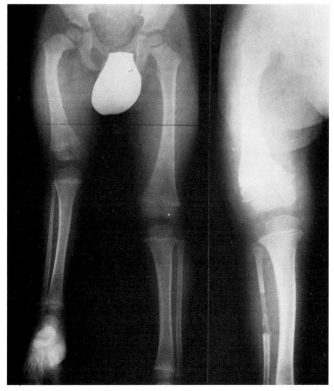

Fig. 3.17 Pre-operative radiograph of congenital short femur showing valgus attitude of the knee and post-operative radiograph after opening wedge osteotomy using a fibular graft.

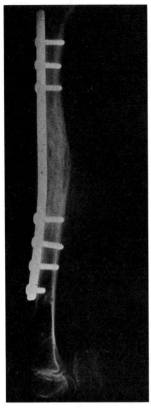

Fig. 3.18 Postoperative radiograph after femoral lengthening. Note that the femur is solid but the tibia has subluxated on the femur.

may prove hazardous to further growth if used in the very young patient, but results in older children may well justify its use in congenital deformities.

Epiphysiodesis. The actual methods of epiphysiodesis have been outlined in the previous discussion under congenital hemihypertrophy and does not present a difficult technical procedure, although tibial epiphysiodesis may also have to be performed.

Summary

The ideal case of the congenital short femur is one of femoral length discrepancy, without the additional problem of an associated distal congenital deficiency. In this situation the treatment planned as outlined should result in a patient with limb length equality with good function having being maintained throughout (Fig. 3.19).

In the situation where there is an associated distal deficiency it is perfectly reasonable to perform a Symes amputation and then, by modest manipulation of the affected femoral segment using the techniques described and epiphysiodesis of the opposite limb, the patient can still enjoy a below knee function with a fairly standard prosthesis. In this situation a significant discrepancy in femoral length can be made up by the prosthetic fitting without significantly detracting from cosmesis or function by a modest discrepancy between the level of the axes of the knees.

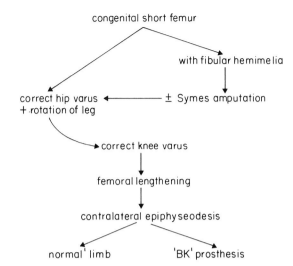

Fig. 3.19 Treatment plan of congenital short femur.

4. Proximal femoral focal deficiency

True PFFD is an uncommon condition, although the management options are reasonably clear and are set out below. Distal femoral focal deficiency, while theoretically possible, has only been reported on one occasion (Tsou 1982).

At first glance, the newborn baby bearing this diagnosis may appear to have a similar deformity to that of the patient with a congenital short femur. Close examination of the infant, however, will reveal differences, although initially subtle, that become more readily apparent with growth.

The clinical features are as follows:

1   The thigh segment is extremely short with the leg in abduction and lateral rotation (Fig. 3.11).
2   There are flexion contractures at both the hip and knee which are fixed and severe and do not resolve with growth (Fig. 3.20).
3   The overall leg length discrepancy is between 35% and 50% with the foot of the affected limb at the level of the contralateral knee (Fig. 3.21).

Although the clinical features are relatively constant, the radiographic appearances of the affected limb show a great variety of deficiencies. The range of these deficiencies has been well illustrated in the classification of Hamanishi (1980). The hypoplasia of the knee joint as shown by the instability in the congenital short femur patient as described previously, is also present in the patient with PFFD. This hypoplasia is seen on X-ray and at surgery. The clinical instability, however, is disguised by the fixed flexion contracture of the knee.

Except in cases of bilateral deficiency, the aim of the surgeon should be to modify the affected limb so as to assist the prosthetist in fitting the patient with an artificial limb which allows both optimal function and cosmesis. The leg is always too short to consider lengthening. The foot appearances vary depending on the presence or absence of an associated terminal deficiency (30–50% have an associated fibular hemimelia). The flexed knee joint provides little, if any, functional value and causes problems in prosthetic fitting. The hip joint although appearing inadequate radiographically in most cases, is nonetheless mobile and painless. Many of these patients have a marked Trendelberg lurch due to lack of femoralpelvic stability and the inadequacy of the abductor mechanism in both bony architecture and the soft tissue muscle bulk. Dissections of the limb have not revealed any muscular anomalies that might be incriminated in the cause of the deformity (Panting & Williams 1978). However, the line of pull of the adductor longus and brevis is seen to be almost at right angles to the line of the femur.

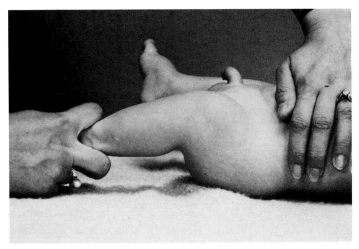

Fig. 3.20 An infant boy with a proximal femoral focal deficiency showing the marked fixed flexion deformities at both hip and knee.

Management

At the initial visit the parents will usually be distressed and want answers to questions which may often surprise the consulting surgeon. With regard to aetiology, a review of cases at the Ontario Crippled Children's Centre (Gillespie

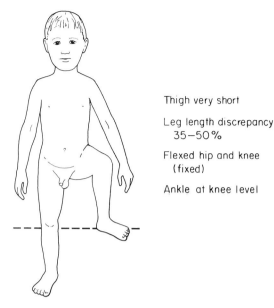

Thigh very short

Leg length discrepancy
35−50%

Flexed hip and knee
(fixed)

Ankle at knee level

Fig. 3.21 Clinical signs of true PFFD.

& Torode 1983) failed to show any hereditary factors although cases of thalidomide ingestion were identified as causing similar deformities to other cases where no such agent could be incriminated (Fig. 3.22). It is important thus to stress that no guilt should be felt by either parent. Secondly, the affected limb can never be made normal and will not be able to be lengthened to a functional length when compared

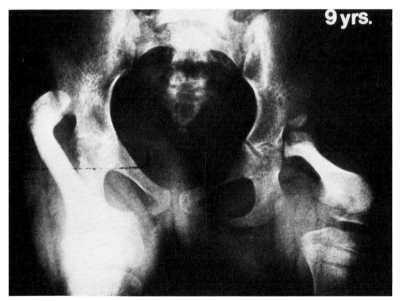

Fig. 3.22 Radiograph of one of twin boys with bilateral marked femoral deficiency secondary to maternal thalidomide ingestion during pregnancy.

to the normal side. Nonetheless, the parents should be made aware of the fact that many patients similarly affected have been known to lead relatively normal lives and are seen to be competent and keen participants in the world of sporting endeavours in which many amputees are involved. Thirdly, decisions regarding surgery can be made early in the life of the child and to delay unnecessarily will only serve to create greater problems both physically and psychologically. Putting off surgical options with the idea that the child should be able to participate in these decisions is not a valid concept.

Surgery

In simple terms, the aim should be to obtain optimal function. The functional value of the foot can be ascertained early in life bearing in mind that a partial deficiency of the foot in association with a fibular hemimelia does not rule out the possibility of a rotationplasty of the below knee segment.

The following surgical and prosthetic programmes are open to the family and patient.

No surgery

The patient will need an extension prosthesis to ambulate as soon as the absolute limb length discrepancy makes walking difficult, even with the foot in as much equinus as possible. Difficulties arise with this option as the flexed knee and hip result in the patient sitting rather than standing in the prosthesis. When the patient adopts this posture it appears that the prosthetic limb is too short, but careful examination will reveal that this is not the case. The lack of stability within the prosthesis is further evidenced by a lurching gait. In some of these patients the limb can be seen pistoning within the prosthesis and there is an associated lack of extension power of the limb as a whole with the functional shortening of the limb further aggravating the gait problem (Fig. 3.23).

Knee fusion — extension prosthesis

If the families of the patients will not consider surgery to the foot of the affected limb then they should be encouraged to consider the benefits of a knee fusion alone. Even if that is the only procedure performed, major benefits in the wearing of the extension prosthesis are gained. The limb within the prosthesis is much more stable. The power transmitted to the prosthesis is greater. The knee flexion contracture is naturally removed at surgery and, following knee fusion, the hip flexion contracture is seen to resolve as well (Fig. 3.24). It should be noted that a knee fusion can be formed as early as the first few years of life as soon as there is a reasonably large distal femoral and proximal tibial epiphysis present. One or both of the associated epiphyseal plates can be retained if thought to be necessary, but usually only the proximal tibial epiphyseal plate is required to provide the necessary limb length for optimal gait with the patient fitted as an effective above-knee wearer.

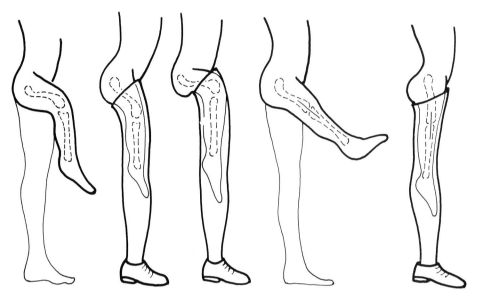

Fig. 3.23 Diagram of prosthetic problems with PFFD, improved by knee fusion.

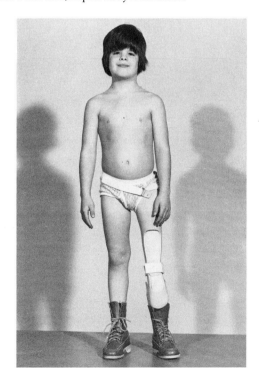

Fig. 3.24 A boy with proximal femoral focal deficiency using an extension prosthesis to equalize leg length.

Knee fusion — Symes amputation — above knee fitting

If the decision has been made not to proceed with a rotationplasty or in situations where there is a significant foot deformity, then retention of the foot serves little purpose. The simplest surgical option to provide optimal function is then a combined early foot ablation and knee fusion. A Symes amputation is done in the routine manner and the knee fusion is performed as described utilizing an intramedullary rod for fixation. One should aim for the stump to be 5–7 cm proximal to the contralateral knee at maturity and thus only the proximal tibial epiphyseal plate needs to be preserved. The end result is that the patient is fitted as an above knee wearer. Prosthetic fitting can be performed only a few weeks after surgery and, once again, the surgical options can be performed early in life allowing the patient to grow and develop often without the need for later surgical procedures. The thigh segment is thus quite long and the often prominent malleoli will provide good suspension for an above knee prosthesis (Figs. 3.25[a] and [b]).

Rotationplasty

While a number of authors have contributed to the orthopaedic literature on the value of tibial rotationplasty (Borgreve 1930, Gillespie & Torode 1983, Kritter 1977) there have been many detractors. To assess the value of this procedure the surgeon should see the functional benefits at first hand before rejecting the concept on emotive grounds (Fisher & Waskowitz 1972).

There are undoubtedly problems with this procedure and these include its timing, derotation of the rotated limb and claims that the limb does not function as intended. These have been addressed by the use of a technique described by Torode and Gillespie (1983). The families should be made aware of the functional benefits of this procedure either by introduction to other patients or by viewing gait videos of patients with prosthetic fitting after rotationplasty (Figs. 3.26[a] and [b]).

Function

When the foot, ankle and tibia have been rotated through 180° and the knee fused, a most functional below-knee fitting is possible. A below-knee amputation has advantages over an above-knee amputation in many areas which include 'knee control', velocity of gait, ability to go up and down steps and reflex action. The reflex adaption of the 'quadriceps' formed by the rotated calf muscles has been identified in the gait laboratory and functionally is of great benefit to the patient (Glynn). This protection against stumbling is certainly not available to an above-knee wearer.

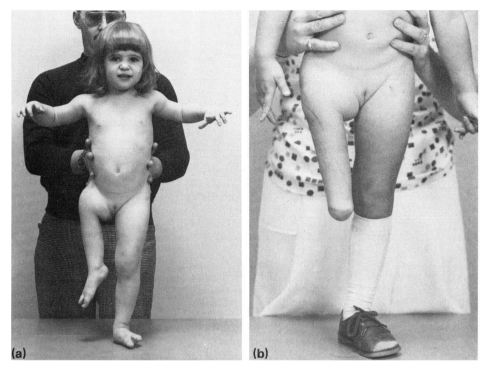

Fig. 3.25 A young girl with a right proximal femoral focal deficiency, (a) pre-operatively and (b) post-operatively having had a knee fusion and Symes amputation performed.

Timing

Just as a knee fusion can be performed, retaining the epiphyseal plates, the modified Van Nes procedure can also be performed at an early age, thus allowing training and adaptation to the limb. Usually the proximal tibial epiphyseal plate is retained and the distal femoral plate removed as this is technically simpler and the amount of growth in the tibia is certainly adequate to provide the appropriate thigh segment length (Figs. 3.27[a], [b] and [c]). In the author's experience, often the limb appears too long in the thigh segment but, on functional grounds, this is not a great problem as the rotated foot has then only to provide power to a relatively short segment which is mechanically less demanding.

Derotation

The problems of derotation have been addressed in a number of papers on this subject. By rotating the tibial segment primarily through the knee joint and by transfer of the medial hamstrings from the tibia to the femur, the problem of muscular torque forces produced by rotating the limb at the midtibial level are avoided (Torode & Gillespie 1983).

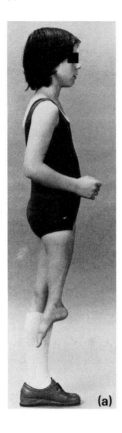 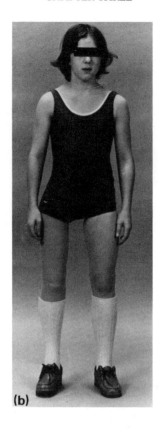

(a) (b)

Fig. 3.26 Showing a teenage girl who has had a Van Nes rotationplasty performed (a) and (b) wearing her prosthesis demonstrating excellent cosmesis.

Foot ablation

In many cases the foot will be deformed and thus no benefit will be gained in its retention. A foot ablation is performed on cosmetic grounds. This procedure is by no means ruled out even when a rotationplasty is thought to be cosmetically unacceptable. The effective end result is thus an above knee wearer as described previously (Fig. 3.25).

Cosmesis

Much has been written about the cosmetic appearance following rotationplasty, yet a review of these cases did not disclose any one patient who wished to have the foot ablated on cosmetic grounds. All the patients were able to appreciate the functional gains of the rotated limb and the retained foot as compared to their peers, who functioned as above knee wearers (Fig. 3.26b).

Hip surgery

There is often a gross deficiency in and around the hip joint of these patients. The

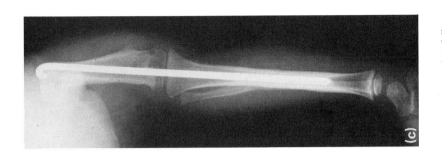

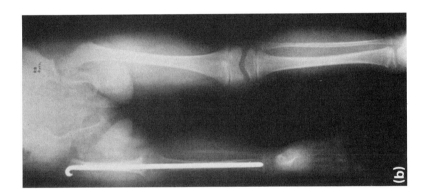

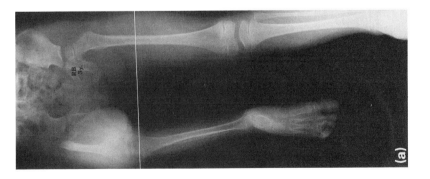

Fig. 3.27 Radiographs of a 3-year-old girl with a PFFD (a) and (b) after Van Nes rotationplasty which has healed and (c) follow-up radiograph showing the open proximal tibial epiphyseal plate. Note the increased distance of the distal end of the rod from the distal tibia illustrating the continued growth of that limb.

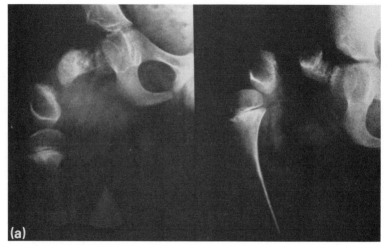

Fig. 3.28(a) Composite radiograph of PFFD patient illustrating the gross instability through the femoral pseudarthrosis.

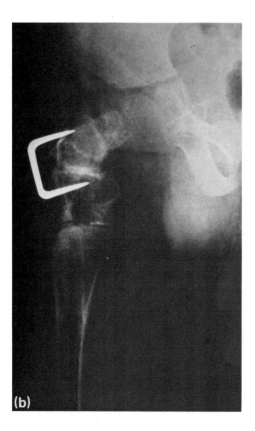

Fig. 3.28(b) Postoperative radiograph with excision of pseudarthrosis and knee fusion.

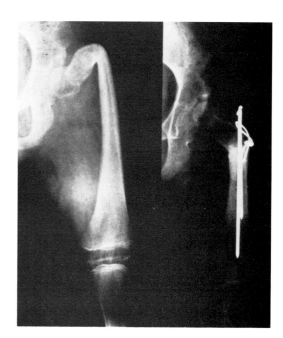

Fig. 3.29 A composite radiograph showing correction of a gross coxa vara of a PFFD patient with abduction osteotomy and knee fusion.

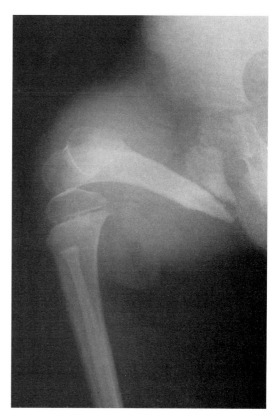

Fig. 3.30 PFFD patient with a gross flexion deformity at the level of the femoral pseudarthrosis.

deficiency is often translated into clinical instability which usually attracts the orthopaedic surgeon's attention (Lane *et al.* 1978). While the radiographic appearances can be improved by surgery to bridge these deficiencies, it is difficult to see what functional gains can be expected. This is partly due to the fact that even though bony continuity is obtained, there remains a deficiency in the abductor mechanism which cannot be overcome. Routine surgical exploration of the hips in these children is not advocated. Clinical examination, radiographs and knowledge of the natural history will provide the information needed.

Indications for surgical intervention at the hip level in PFFD are:

1   To stabilize the hip where gross instability exists through a pseudarthrosis (Figs. 3.28[a] and [b]).
2   To correct and prevent progression of gross coxa vara (Fig. 3.29).
3   To correct a major flexion deformity at the level of a pseudarthrosis (Fig. 3.30).
4   To prevent pain and skin breakdown due to pressure from proximal migration of a spindle shaped upper end of the distal femoral fragment.

Summary

The unilateral PFFD patient presents problems of a gross limb length deformity that will require prosthetic management. There are surgical procedures available which will enhance both cosmesis and function. These procedures can be performed early in life and thus allow early adaptation and prosthetic fitting. In the first few years of life, the surgeon should outline the surgical plans available to the families concerned and a decision should be made as to whether above-knee or below-knee function will be the goal (Fig. 3.31). In bilateral cases, each situation must be treated

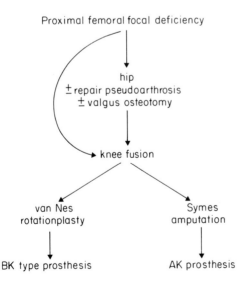

Proximal femoral focal deficiency

hip
± repair pseudoarthrosis
± valgus osteotomy

knee fusion

van Nes
rotationplasty

Symes
amputation

BK type prosthesis

AK prosthesis

Fig. 3.31 Treatment plan of true PFFD patient.

on its merits. Bilateral extension prostheses have been fitted to some patients in order to obtain standing height in social circumstances but most patients discard these because they inhibit their mobility. Variable bilateral involvement is sometimes seen where one lower limb would come under the classifications of congenital short femur and the other limb a true proximal femoral focal deficiency and in these situations the plan of action would depend on the relative length of both limbs. It is difficult to imagine the need to perform a lengthening in the congenital short femur in this situation, although the PFFD limb may justify treatment along similar lines as for a unilateral PFFD.

References

Aitken G. T. (1969) *Proximal Femoral Focal Deficiency — Definition, Classification, and Management In Proximal Femoral Focal Deficiency.* A Congenital Anomaly, 1–22. National Academy of Sciences, Washington D. C.

Almond H. G. (1956) Familial infantile coxa vara. *Journal of Bone and Joint Surgery,* **38B,** 539–44.

Alsberg A. (1899) Theory and differential diagnosis of coxa vara. *Zeitschrift für Orthopädische Chirurgie,* **7,** 365.

Amstutz H. C. & Wilson P.D. Jr. (1962) Dysgenesis of the proximal femur (coxa vara) and its surgical management. *Journal of Bone and Joint Surgery,* **44A,** 1–23.

Anderson M., Green W. T. & Messner M. B. (1963) Growth and predictions of growth in the lower extremities. *Journal of Bone and Joint Surgery,* **45A,** 1–14.

Anderson M. & Green W. T. (1948) Lengths of the femur and the tibia. *American Journal of Diseases of Children,* **75,** 279–90.

Babb F. S., Ghormley R. & Chatterton C. C. (1949) Congenital coxa vara. *Journal of Bone and Joint Surgery,* **31A,** 115–31.

Bell J. S. & Thompson W. A. (1950) Modified spot scanography. *American Journal of Roentgenology,* **63,** 915–16.

Binazzi R. Personal communications.

Blount W. P. (1949) Trauma and growing bones. *Septieme Congres de la Société Internationale de Chirurgine Orthopedique et de Traumatologie.* Barcelona.

Blount W. P. & Clark G. R. (1949) Control of bone growth by epiphyseal stapling. Preliminary report. *Journal of Bone and Joint Surgery,* **31A,** 464–78.

Borgreve J. (1930) Kniegelenksersatz durch das in der Beinlangsachse um 180⁰ gedrehte Fussglenk. *Archir für orthopädische und Unfall-Chirurgie,* **28,** 175–8.

Bryan R. S., Lipscomb P. R. & Chatterton C. C. (1958) Orthopaedic aspects of congenital hemihypertrophy. *American Journal of Surgery,* **96,** 654–659.

Canale S. T., Russell T. A. & Holcomb R. L. (1986) Percutaneous epiphyseodesis — experimental study and preliminary clinical results. *Journal of Pediatric Orthopedics,* **6(2),** 150–6.

Cowell H. R. (1978) *Pediatric Orthopedics* (Lovell & Winter eds) Vol. 1, Chap. 5 J. B. Lippincott and Co., Philadelphia.

Fiorani G. (1948) quoted by Zadek I. Congenital coxa vara. *Archives of Surgery,* **30,** 62.

Fisher R. L. & Waskowitz W. J. (1972) Familial development coxa vara. *Clinical Orthopaedics and Related Research,* **86,** 2–5.

Fixsen J. A. (1983) Rotation plasty. *Journal of Bone and Joint Surgery,* **65B,** 529.

Fixsen J. A. & Lloyd-Roberts G. C. (1974) The natural history and early treatment of proximal femoral dysplasia. *Journal of Bone and Joint Surgery,* **56B,** 86–95.

Gillespie R. & Torode I. (1983) Classification and management of congenital deficiences of the lower limbs. *Journal of Bone and Joint Surgery,* **65B,** 557–68.

Glynn M. Investigation into gait pattern and muscle function following V.N. rotation osteotomy in PFFD. OCCC, Toronto, Canada. Unpublished.

Goff C. W. (1960) Surgical treatment of unequal extremities. Charles C. Thomas, Springfield, Illinois.

Golding F. C. (1948) Congenital coxa vara. *Journal of Bone and Joint Surgery*, **30B**, 161–3.

Green W. T. & Anderson M. (1947) Experiences with epiphyseal arrest in correcting discrepancies in length of the lower extremities in infantile paralysis. *Journal of Bone and Joint Surgery*, **29A**, 659–75.

Green W. T. & Anderson M. (1955) The problem of unequal leg lengths. *Paediatric Clinics of North America*, **2**, 1137–1155.

Green W. T. & Anderson M. (1960) Skeletal age and control of bone growth. *American Association of Orthopaedic Surgeons Instructional Course Lectures*, **17**, 199–217.

Green W. T., Wyatt G. M. & Anderson M. (1946) Orthoroentgenography as a method of measuring bones of the lower extremities. *Journal of Bone and Joint Surgery*, **28B**, 60–65.

Greulich W. W. & Pyle S. I. (1959) *Radiographic atlas of Skeletal Development of the Hand and Wrist*, second edition. Stanford University Press.

Hamanishi C. (1980) Congenital short femur. *Journal of Bone and Joint Surgery*, **62B**, 307–20.

Helms C. A. C. T. (1984) Scanograms for measuring leg length discrepancy. *Radiology*, **151(3)**, 802.

Hoffa A. (1905) Congenital coxa vara. *Deutsche medizinische Wochenschrift*, **31**, 1257.

Hofmeister (1949) quoted by Babb F. S. *et al.* Congenital coxa vara. *Journal of Bone and Joint Surgery*, **31A**, 115–131.

Hensinger R. N. & Jones T. (1981) *Neonatal Orthopaedics*. Grune and Stratton, New York.

Jones D. C. & Moseley C. F. (1985) Subluxation of the knee as a complication of femoral lengthening by the Wagner technique. *Journal of Bone and Joint Surgery*, **67B**, 33–5.

Kritter A. E. (1977) Tibial rotation-plasty for proximal femoral focal deficiency. *Journal of Bone and Joint Surgery*, **59A**, 927–34.

Lange D. R., Schoenecker P. L. & Baker C. L. (1978) PFFD treatment and classification in 42 cases. *Clinical Orthopaedics and Related Research*, **135**, 15–25.

Marchetti P. G. & Faldini A. (1968) *Il Trattamento Chirurgico della Coxa Vara*. Carlo Erba,

Menelaus M. B. (1966) Correction of leg length discrepancy by epiphyseal arrest. *Journal of Bone and Joint Surgery*, **48B**, 336–339.

Mezhenina E. P., Roulla E. A., Pecherusky A. G., Babich V. D., Shadrina E. L. & Mizhevich T. V. (1984) Methods of limb elongation with congenital inequality in children. *Journal of Paediatric Orthopaedics*, **4(2)**, 201–7.

Morris J. V. & MacGillivray R. C. (1955) Mental defects and hemihypertrophy. *American Journal of Mental Deficieny*, **59**, 645–51.

Moseley C. F. (1977) A straight line graph for leg length discrepancies. *Journal of Bone and Joint Surgery*, **59A**, 174–9.

Nilsonne H. (1928) On congenital coxa vara. *Acta chirurgica Scandinavia*, **64**, 217–28.

Ogilvie J. W. (1986) Epiphyseodesis: evaluation of a new technique. *Journal of Paediatric Orthopaedics*, **6(2)**, 147–9.

Panting A. L. & Williams P. F. (1978) Proximal focal femoral deficieny. *Journal of Bone and Joint Surgery*, **60B**, 46–52.

Pauwels F. (1976) *Biomechanics of the Normal and Disabled*. H. P. Springer Verlag, Berlin.

Phemister D. B. (1933) Operative arrest of longitudinal growth of bones in treatment of deformities. *Journal of Bone and Joint Surgery*, **15**, 1–15.

Pyllkanen P. V. (1960) Coxa vara infantum. *Acta orthopaedica Scandinavica*, **48 (Supp)**, 1–120.

Salai W., Chechick A., Ganel A., Blankstein A., Horoszowski H. (1985) Subluxation of the hip during femoral lengthening. *Journal of Paediatric Orthopaedics*, **5:6**, 642–4.

Scott A. J. (1935) Hemihypertrophy. Report of 4 cases. *Journal of Paediatrics*, **6**, 650–6.

Tachdjian M. (1982) *Paediatric Orthopaedics*. W. B. Saunders Co., Philadelphia.

Temtamy S. & Rogers J. G. (1976) Macrodactyly, hemihypertrophy and connective tissue nevi. Report of a new syndrome. *Journal of Paediatrics*, **89:6**, 924–7.

Torode I. & Gillespie R. (1983) Anteroposterior instability of the knee. *Journal of Paediatric Orthopaedics*, **3**: 467–70.

Torode I. & Gillespie R. (1983) Tibial rotationplasty in PFFD. *Journal of Bone and Joint Surgery*, **65B**, 569–78.

Tsou P. L. (1982) Congenital distal focal femoral deficiency. *Clinical Orthopaedics and Related Research* **162**, 99–102.

Van Nes C. P. (1950) Rotationplasty for congenital defects of the femur. Making use of the ankle of the shortened limb to control the knee joint of a prosthesis. *Journal of Bone and Joint Surgery,* **32B,** 12–16.

Wagner H. (1839) Hypertrophie der rechten Brust und der rechten Oberen Extremität besonders der Hand und der Finger. *Med. Jahrb. d. k. k. Österreichischen Staates,* **19,** 378.

Wagner H. (1971) Operative Beinver. angerung. Der Chirug. **42(6),** 260–

Ward J. & Lerner H., (1947) A review of the subject of hemihypertrophy. *Journal of Paediatrics,* **31,** 403–14.

Weinstein J. N., Kuo K. N. & Millar E. A. (1984) Congenital coxa vara — a retrospective view. *Journal of Paediatric Orthopaedics,* **4(1),** 70–77.

White J. W. & Stubbins S. G. Jr. (1944) Growth arrest for equalizing leg lengths. *Journal of the Australian Medical Association,* **126,** 1146–49.

Williams J. A. (1951) Congenital hemihypertrophy with lymphangioma. *Archives of Disease in Childhood,* **26,** 158–61.

Winquist R. A., Hansen S. T. Jr. & Pearson R. E. (1978) Closed intramedullary shortening of the femur. *Clinical Orthopaedics and Related Research,* **136,** 54–61.

Zadek I. (1935) Congenital coxa vara. *Archives of Surgery,* **30,** 62–102.

4

Congenital Dislocation of the Hip

M. F. MACNICOL

Introduction

One of the peculiarities of orthopaedics in childhood is the fact that the hip joint, which normally functions in the adult as a highly stable ball and socket articulation, is very prone to displacement in the first years of life. This chapter examines the implications of that clinical conundrum by reviewing the management of the condition during the different stages of childhood. The nature of the problem is greatly influenced by the age of the child at presentation since progressive delay in securing a precise and durable reduction assuredly destroys the hip before its time.

A serious difficulty in understanding the reasons behind the management of this idiopathic displacement stems from a confusion in terminology. For instance, the clinical difference between a clicking hip at birth and a genuine instability of the joint is not always appreciated. Furthermore, there is uncertainty about the relationship between neonatal hip instability and subsequent displacement of the hip, and the use of the terms dysplasia, preluxation, subluxation and dislocation implies a continuum of pathological changes to some orthopaedic surgeons, while to others these words are now considered to be neither accurate not interrelated. Additionally, the prognosis for each hip after an apparently satisfactory reduction is difficult to predict and hence there is great divergence of opinion about the type and timing of surgical procedures in the toddler. The adequacy of acetabular growth is obviously of paramount importance, yet there is no certain method by which this may by ensured.

As a result of these uncertainties an enormous variation in the incidence of neonatal and juvenile displacement of the hip is presented in the orthopaedic literature. Racial and geographical differences also have to be considered, for they undoubtedly affect both the frequency and severity of hip dysplasia and dislocation encountered throughout the world. Finally, methods of conservative and operative management of the abnormal hip are universally uncontrolled and subject to highly individualistic bias such that attempts at interpreting results proves to be a frustrating venture. Surgical complications need to be reported fully since they influence the future of the patient as much as the adequacy of reduction. The penalties incurred by the child from femoral head ischaemia, from pressure deformities with resultant incongruities within the joint, and from poorly executed pelvic and femoral osteotomies, are indeed severe and may overshadow the intended benefits of surgical treatment.

The consequences of untreated displacement

Untreated cases of subluxation or dislocation of the hip are asymptomatic initially. However, the growth abnormality and articular cartilage damage which ensue lead to an irreversible decline in joint function. This is not to say that the hip will cease to bear weight since high, bilateral dislocations regularly permit an active and relatively pain free life, at least until middle age. But the abnormal stresses produce capsular pain, muscle spasm as a protective response, and eventually backache and knee symptoms. Gradually the restrictive action of the hip muscles proves inadequate, such that a subluxation will progress, despite contractures and the remarkable hypertrophy of the round ligament, capsule and the reflected head of the rectus femoris.

Although pain is first perceived during exertion, symptoms develop at rest as arthritic changes occur between any areas of articular cartilage which remain in contact. In addition to the cardinal symptom of pain, which is felt in the groin, diffusely over the proximal thigh and in the knee, the hip gradually stiffens and may click or give way. Leg length is decreased to a variable extent, depending on the degree of real and apparent shortening, and gait worsens appreciably.

Possible aetiological factors

In the typical case of neonatal hip instability (Table 4.1) the position of the fetus *in utero* and the subsequent events at the time of birth are of great significance. An extended breech position prior to delivery (Wilkinson 1963 & 1985) or a prolonged and difficult labour will force the hips into extension. This in turn will promote a displacement of the femoral head which may be temporary or permanent. The acetabulum, although recognizably cup-shaped and formed from the triradiate cartilage linking the ilium, ischium and pubis (Fig. 4.1), is nevertheless significantly reliant upon the labrum (Fig. 4.2) for the provision of a strong hold upon the femoral head. Capsular strength, muscle tone and a negative intra-articular pressure further resist movement of the femoral head away from the acetabulum.

Carter and Wilkinson (1964) hypothesized that temporary laxity of the hip at the time of childbirth resulted from the effects of maternal hormones, particularly raised levels of oestrone and progesterone. Relaxin, a polypeptide produced by the oestrogen-sensitive uterus in response to progesterone, was also considered to be contributory, possibly explaining the female predominance of hip instability in the neonatal period. On the other hand, permanent joint laxity appears to be

Table 4.1 Typical and atypical forms of congenital displacement of the hip.

Typical	neonatal instability
	infantile dysplasia ('preluxation')
	infantile subluxation
	infantile dislocation
	juvenile subluxation (possibly primary)
Atypical	principally the rare 'teratological' forms (teratos = monster)
	associated with arthrogryposis, myelodysplasias, gross hypotonias
	and major chromomosal defects

genetically determined with an incidence of 1 or 2 per 100, and is probably responsible for later presentation of familial hip dislocation (Wynne-Davies 1970a).

Bado (1963) emphasized the importance of neuromuscular mechanisms which are known to play such a pivotal role in determining hip stability in cerebral palsy, spina bifida and allied neurological disorders. It may well be that certain forms of

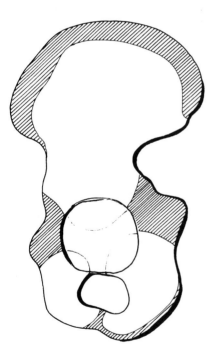

Fig. 4.1 The acetabulum is formed centrally by the triradiate cartilage which links the ossifying contiguous portions of the ilium, ischium and pubis.

'typical' congenital displacement of the hip are secondary to a persistent imbalance in muscle power around the hip or in the tonic reflexes which govern posture. This may in part explain the increased incidence of dislocation in children with a skeletal skew that includes pelvic obliquity and scoliosis.

Monticelli and Milella (1982) promoted the concept, already alluded to in 1963 by Mitchell, that certain dislocated hips are lax or loose, whereas others are tight and therefore difficult to reduce, possibly because of 'muscular tension'.

Pathological increases in the relative strength and tone of the psoas, adductors and rectus femoris were considered by them to be particularly important, such that treatment would fail if a balance is not restored by means of muscle releases and transfers (similar to the concepts adhered to in treating club foot). In those children with significant muscle imbalance, not only is reduction more difficult to maintain, but ischaemic damage to the femoral head is more readily incurred and the effects of rotation femoral osteotomy, in particular, may be negated or even reversed by the persistent deformation produced by unbalanced muscle forces.

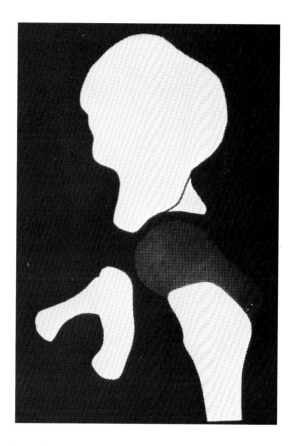

Fig. 4.2 This anteroposterior projection shows how the labrum deepens the acetabulum by encompassing the equator of the femoral head. Note that the proximal femur is composed entirely of cartilage in the young infant.

Neonatal screening for the unstable hip

Roser (1864) first realised that it was possible to diagnose instability of the hip in the newborn, producing dislocation by adducting the legs and relocation by abducting the legs. Le Damany introduced a systematic examination of the hips in the neonate at La Maternité in Paris and in Rennes, publishing his findings in 1912. He did not touch upon the possibility of a relationship between neonatal laxity, which he considered to be self-limiting, and late dislocation. Le Damany's sign of 'ressaut' and Ortolani's 'segno del scatto' (1948) both describe the jolt, clunk or gliding over a ridge that characterize the sense of dislocation as the femoral head moves backwards and forwards over the labrum.

Putti (1933) and Marx (1938) maintained the European interest in neonatal hip instability, but the real boost to this endeavour arose from the publications of Palmén (1961) and von Rosen (1962) in Sweden. Screening of the neonate began in 1950 and was found to influence the incidence of late dislocation.

The incidence of hip instability at birth varies greatly, with rates in the UK of between 1 in 60 live births (Barlow 1962) and 1 in 250 live births (Macnicol 1985). Racial differences are even more marked, with 1 in 5 hips reported as abnormal in North American Indians, high rates in Eastern Europe and the Mediterranean, yet only 1 in 1000 in the Chinese and virtually none in African Negroes (Tachdjian 1982). If high-pitched clicks are excluded, in the belief that these emanate from the iliotibial tract and from ligaments, then true instability probably only occurs in approximately 1 in 200 infants. The clunk is perceived as a feeling rather than as a sound, although, as with the McMurray rotation test for a torn meniscus in the knee, it may also be audible. Clinical examination should reveal either an exit clunk, by pushing posteriorly with the hip adducted (Barlow's test [1962] or the 'subluxation by provocation' test of Andrén [1961; Fig. 4.3]), or an entry clunk by lifting the femoral head forward into the socket with circumduction and forward pressure upon the greater trochanter (Ortolani's manoeuvre [1948]; Fig. 4.4).

More than half of these unstable hips become normal to clinical examination during the first week or two of life. All that remain displaced will present in later life as a dislocated hip, while a proportion of the dislocateable hips will lead on to dislocation or subluxation in later childhood. It may well be that some hips which appear clinically normal at birth will give rise to problems at walking age although this group is small, perhaps 0.2 to 0.6 per 1000 live births. However, the significance of this incidence of 'missed' cases increases if the natural incidence of the condition is considered to be low. Thus Record and Edwards (1958) found that in the Manchester area of England the incidence of true, late-presenting congenital dislocation of the hip was 0.6 per 1000 children, at a time when screening was not in force. However, the more generally accepted late incidence of hip dislocation in Caucasians is 1.5 per 1000, and if this estimate is still applicable today, at least two out of every three cases of potentially irreversible hip dispacement are prevented by screening at birth and early splintage (Macnicol 1985; Dunn *et al.* 1985).

The incidence of late dislocation and subluxation is also racially determined, with high rates in Japan, the Mediterranean and Eastern Europe. American Indians present commonly with the condition (Coleman 1978), and this was partly the result of the use of a cradle board or 'tikanogen' during infancy. The legs of these infants were held relatively immobile in extension and adduction, but fortunately this cultural practice is now discouraged.

The prevention of late presentation should continue to be the aim of effective neonatal screening programmes, despite the disappointments encountered by certain regions in the UK (Mackenzie & Wilson 1981, Catford *et al.* 1982) where

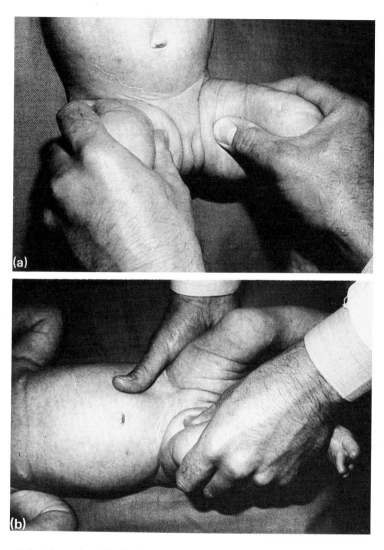

Fig. 4.3 An exit clunk is produced in the dislocateable hip by pushing the proximal femur posteriorly with the thumb, either with both hands placed on the thighs as shown in (a) or by stabilizing the pelvis with one hand as shown in (b).

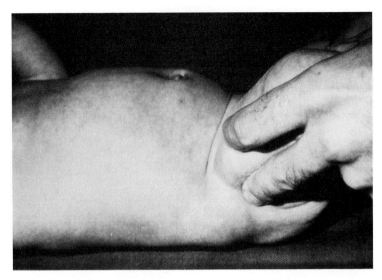

Fig. 4.4 The dislocated hip is identified by the entry clunk produced by lifting the greater trochanter forwards with the middle finger. Circumduction or abduction may also reduce the hip with a palpable jolt or clunk.

the incidence of dislocation in childhood has been unaffected by examination and treatment of the hips at birth.

Although the main preoccupation is with neonatal screening, improvements in community medical care and regular inspection of the child before walking age have changed the pattern of later presentation (Palmén 1984) such that more infants with suspicious hips are being referred between the ages of three and twelve months. These cases may represent missed diagnoses at birth. But it is clear that some have been carefully examined in maternity units by experienced examiners, and yet do not manifest until later. Despite this sobering fact, the importance of neonatal screening by enthusiastic and trained personnel should not be diminished. The efficiency of screening now depends upon paediatricians, health visitors and general practitioners to a greater extent than upon the orthopaedic surgeon, and their combined interest and teamwork relies upon close cooperation and regular communication with those whose commitment includes the management of the child with an established dislocation.

Factors associated with neonatal hip displacement are shown in Table 4.2 and Fig. 4.5. These should alert the examiner who follows a strict routine when examining the newborn:

1   The infant should be relaxed, warm and preferably quiet; the best time to examine the hip is therefore after a feed when the baby is in a nursery or at the mother's bedside.
2   The nappy should be removed and the infant placed upon a firm surface, such as a cot board with a folded blanket upon its surface.

Table 4.2 Neonatal factors associated with hip displacement.

Exogenous	Female (75% of cases)
	First-born child (50% of cases)
	Family history of hip dislocation (10% of cases)
	Breech position, difficult labour or Caesarean section
	Oligohydramnios
	Maternal hypertension
Endogenous	Plagiocephaly or torticollis
	Scoliosis
	Skeletal skew
	Foot deformity (calcaneovalgus, metatarsus adductus, equinovarus)
	Umbilical or other herniae
	Skin pigmentation or hairy patches

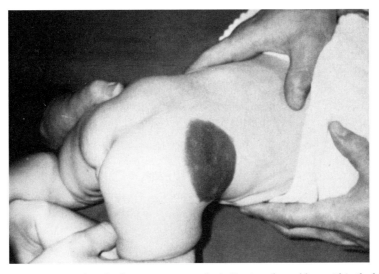

Fig. 4.5 Skin blemishes, such as this large naevus, may be indicative of a problem within the hip joint.

3   The examiner may either sit or stand, and should assess each hip in turn, after first checking
   (a) the skull for asymmetry
   (b) the upper limbs
   (c) the spine and pelvis for asymmetry
   (d) the knees and the feet
4   There is no set routine for assessing the hips, but physical examination should include:
   (a) a review of the symmetry of the thighs, of active movements and of the presence or absence of the normal, infantile hip flexion deformity.
   (b) a careful measure of the passive range of movements in each hip, particularly abduction in flexion.

(c) an attempt to dislocate the femoral head posteriorly by holding the thigh in the hand as shown (Fig. 4.3), so that the thumb presses against the inner aspect of the proximal thigh; the knee should be held fully flexed in order to relax the iliotibial tract and thus reduce the chance of producing a ligamentous click; the exit clunk of a dislocatable hip is more readily precipitated if the thigh is adducted, and the posterior movement may be sufficient to cause the fleshy thigh to shake; a better perception of the clunk is afforded if the opposite hand is placed behind the pelvis.

(d) a check that the femoral head is not lying in a dislocated position by attempting to produce an entry clunk, pulling forwards with the middle finger on the greater trochanter (Fig. 4.4); this test may not invariably disclose a dislocation, particularly if there is an unyielding obstruction to reduction.

Each examiner develops a technique that should become familiar and should incorporate the steps detailed above. Limitation of abduction and asymmetry should alert the clinician as much as the presence of a clunk, and if there is any doubt, the infant should be re-examined later that day. A further examination is ensured prior to discharge home, and a second opinion should always be sought when there is any doubt about the diagnosis. An effective screening programme is a team effort above all, with cooperation between paediatric, orthopaedic and nursing staff initially, and the community medical services later.

Radiography

In cases where the diagnosis remains in doubt, or when there is a strong family history of congenital dislocation of the hip, a standardized anteroposterior pelvic radiograph is of some value. It is impractical to investigate all babies in this manner, but in suspicious cases, including those where asymmetry suggests a skeletal deformation or fetopathy (Dunn 1976), carefully taken films add to the precision of neonatal screening (Bertol *et al.* 1982).

Radiographic assessment of the unstable hip was first considered by Le Damany (1912) and considerably refined by Andrén (1961) who suggested that X-rays of the hips be obtained with the legs both in the neutral position (patellae pointing forwards) and in abduction with internal rotation of 45°. Pelvic 'instability' secondary to ligament laxity can also be demonstrated radiographically by stress films with the abducted legs pushed together and then pulled apart (Andrén 1962), although the application of this technique is very limited and open to considerable misinterpretation.

The use of neonatal radiographs is controversial, but properly executed films at a set focal distance from the infant can be measured reliably. Scrutiny of the data used to refute the value of this investigation invariably shows it to be anecdotal rather than systematic, and careful statistical analysis (Bertol, *et al.* 1982) has shown that not only the unstable hip but also its contralateral, and apparently normal, partner 'stand off' laterally with an increase in the medial gap. As this occurs, the proximal femur also moves progressively superiorly (Figs. 4.6 & 4.7).

The major drawback in the use of radiographs is that only those hips considered to be clinically abnormal are subjected to this investigation, and therefore it does not prevent cases from being missed in the group without an X-ray. This is a serious limitation and it must be appreciated that radiographs can only improve the accuracy of diagnosis in babies with suspicious hips. The importance of technical precision in producing these films is also acknowledged for they cannot be interpreted when artefacts such as pelvic rotation (Tonnis 1976) and leg position are uncontrolled. It has been proposed that radiographs of all children be obtained later in the first year of life, perhaps at six or nine months of age. Regrettably, the assessment of the pelvic radiograph at this later stage in development may not prove any more advantageous since the degree of ossification of the capital femoral epiphysis is extremely variable (Bertol *et al.* 1982) and the same positional artefacts are operant.

Ultrasound

This investigation is noninvasive and gives a dynamic portrayal of the hip joint and of any soft tissue distortions. The equipment consists of an advanced technology sector scanner which produces a three-dimensional display from two projected views. The scanner is portable and the results of examination can be stored and reviewed at a later date. While the application of ultrasound promises to improve the precision of diagnosis (Clark *et al.* 1985) there is still the logistical problem of scanning every hip at birth. If only those hips that arouse clinical suspicion are examined, then, as with radiography, there will be a small cohort of apparently normal children where instability of the hip may pass unnoticed.

Treatment at birth

Barlow (1962) pointed out that over half the hips that he considered to be unstable at birth became clinically normal in the first few weeks of life, and that as many as 80% will do so by the age of two months. The problem is that there is no means of predicting at birth which hip will remain unstable, although the joint presenting with an entry clunk, particularly if bilateral, is more likely to remain displaced than the hip with an intermittent exit clunk. Furthermore, many mothers are admitted nowadays on a '48-hour discharge' basis, and the hips cannot therefore be reassessed over an extended period of time. Fortunately, the frequency of hip instability does not appear to be greater than 3–6 per 1000, and therefore a policy of splintage can be pursued for this group of infants without incurring the charge that unnecessarily large numbers of babies are being treated. If greater numbers of infants do receive treatment then one must seriously consider whether the screening process is itself breeding a syndrome which is of no consequence in

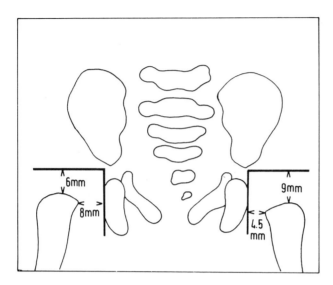

Fig. 4.6 A well-centred anteroposterior pelvic radiograph taken at a focal distance of 1 metre reveals any displacement of the hip by an enlargement of the 'medial gap' between the ossified proximal femur and the ischium (up to 4.5 mm normally), and a corresponding decrease in the superior gap. The legs should not be abducted as this may reduce the unstable hip; instead, the thighs are held parallel with the trunk with the patellae pointing anteriorly.

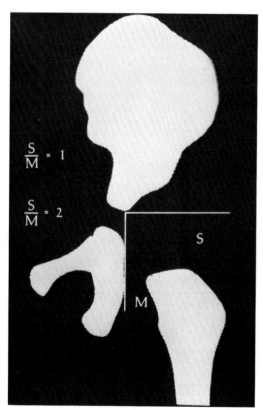

Fig. 4.7 In the unstable hip the ratio of the superior gap to the medial gap (S/M) therefore approaches 1, whereas the normal value for S/M is 2.

relation to the later well-being of the hips.

For the dislocateable hip with an exit clunk, or the readily reducible hip, a Pavlik harness (Pavlik 1957) is recommended for two or three months respectively. The splint (Fig. 4.8) should be applied by an experienced clinician, physiotherapist or orthotist, and is rechecked regularly. A pelvic radiograph at one month of age, with the harness in place, ensures that the hips are reduced. The stability of the hips can also be assessed by establishing the position of the greater trochanters by palpation. A hip that tends to dislocate posteriorly in spite of flexion and moderate abduction, and this is best assessed by checking the stability of the greater

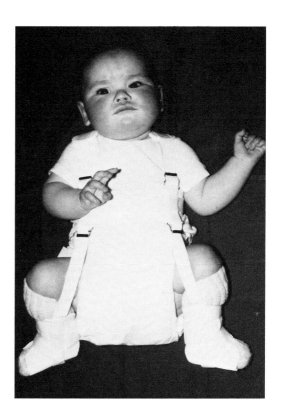

Fig. 4.8 The Pavlik harness maintains the legs in 45–60° of abduction and approximately 90° of flexion. The straps should be adjusted intermittently to preserve this position and a bulky nappy supports the abduction.

trochanters, may be controlled more effectively by a loosely applied Malmo splint (Fig. 4.9). Both types of splint are retained day and night for two or three months, and the mother must be conversant with the restrictions in bathing and clothing the baby before she leaves the hospital. If a health visitor, district nurse or a 'mothers' club' can offer help at home, then the difficulties in nursing the baby are very much lessened. No psychological or physical harm to the baby results, and bonding between a splinted infant and the mother seems to be unaffected.

The risks of producing a pressure (ischaemic) necrosis of the proximal femoral epiphysis or growth plate are very slight with the Pavlik harness, perhaps 0.5–1.0%.

Excessive flexion of the hips must be avoided as this may injure the femoral nerve. Therefore the straps of the harness should be lengthened as the baby grows, and careful supervision of the splint during its use over several months may have to be ensured by the orthopaedic surgeon, physiotherapist or district nurse. Equally, the harness must not be allowed to loosen appreciably since its therapeutic effect will be lost.

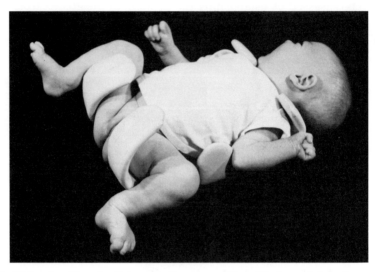

Fig. 4.9 The Malmo (von Rosen) splint secures the same position of flexion and abduction and the nappy is placed behind the splint both posteriorly and anteriorly. Note that the lower struts allow the thighs to move freely from approximately 60 to 90° of abduction.

The Malmo splint is an extremely effective splint, but more cumbersome. It is therefore less acceptable to some mothers although infants settle into it well if the upper struts are properly adjusted over the shoulders and away from the neck. Perhaps surprisingly, a proportion of the parents prefer the more rigid structure of the Malmo splint to the rather fiddly buckles and straps of the Pavlik harness. Since using a loose Malmo splint with a nappy to control the legs within the lower struts, there have been no cases of proximal femoral cartilage injury in Edinburgh (Bertol *et al.* 1982).

After one month of splintage, the position of the legs within the splint should be checked at a clinic. A radiograph will confirm whether the hips are reduced at this stage. For the remaining one or two months of splintage, the Pavlik harness is usually sufficient, and its use can be continued full-time or during the night for approximately a further six months if the hips still give cause for concern. However, the recurrence of a dislocation after apparently satisfactory splintage suggests that an obstruction is present within the joint (Fig. 4.10).

Alternative splints, such as the Craig (Aberdeen) splint and Frejka pillow, are placed over the nappy and are inevitably removed regularly during the day. The more unstable hip may be allowed to displace and the results of treatment are therefore less certain than with the Malmo and Pavlik devices which produce normal hip development in close to 100% of cases (Fredensborg 1977, Dunn *et al.* 1985). Double nappies, even reinforced by prone lying, cannot exert sufficient control over an unstable hip and therefore any hip with a proven exit or entry clunk merits formal splintage. Fixed and forced positions of abduction and flexion must be avoided, however, and it is better not to have treated the hips at all at this age than to produce serious deformation of the upper femur.

The principal complications of management in the neonatal period are therefore:

1 missed diagnosis;
2 failures of splintage;
3 iatrogenic pressure lesions of the femoral head and growth plate.

The rate of diagnostic error varies greatly (Bennet *et al.* 1982, Dunn *et al.* Fredensborg 1977, Mackenzie & Wilson 1981, Macnicol 1985) and may have increased since the earlier results of screening (von Rosen 1962, Mitchell 1972).

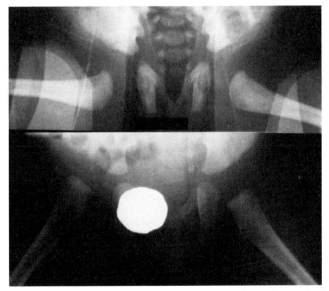

Fig. 4.10 In spite of a satisfactory reduction radiograph in the Malmo splint (top), the right hip subsequently dislocated and the left acetabulum has developed poorly (2 months later.)

However, an efficient programme should be able to pick up and treat effectively at least two out of every three hips that might otherwise present late, thus reducing the late diagnosis rate from approximately 1.5 per 1000 to 0.5 per 1000.

Failures of the splint to retain the femoral head in the acetabulum are rare, perhaps 1 or 2%, although on occasions it will be found that a commercial splint will not secure reduction. In those cases, a few weeks in a carefully moulded spica may be required although there is an appreciable risk of producing ischaemic changes in the proximal femur. This last, and iatrogenic, complication of early treatment can largely be avoided by positioning the legs physiologically and by gentle handling of the infant.

Treatment during infancy (3–12 months)

Although the ideal age for treatment is during the first week of life, diagnosis and careful treatment at a later stage in the first year of life is still to be preferred to a presentation after the child is walking. However precarious the vascularity of the femoral head, careful reduction is recommended as soon as possible. Therefore, although it may be appropriate to delay treatment until the tenth or twelfth month in a small proportion of cases (Mitchell 1983), it is recommended that mobile splintage be used after closed or open reduction, which should in turn follow preliminary traction and the precision afforded by videoarthrography.

Palmén (1984) has described how those hips 'missed' at birth are now being referred at an earlier age for orthopaedic treatment. The increasing vigilance and training of community medical personnel is resulting in many more cases being diagnosed secondarily at 4–8 months of age, rather than at 18 months of age or older. Furthermore, there is some evidence to suggest that the later presentation of a dysplastic or dislocated hip may reflect, not so much an inadequate neonatal examination, but the development of a measurable, clinical abnormality only some time after birth. Hence screening of the hips both at birth and later in the first year of life is mandatory.

In addition to the group of hips that present *de novo* at this period there is a small number who have not responded to neonatal splintage. The crucial finding on physical examination is not the presence of hip instability, although this may still be discerned in the child with ligament laxity, but a reduced range of hip movement. A common confusion occurs in an intermediate group of infants in whom the total range of movement is equivalent in each hip but where the arcs differ in relation to the long axis of the body. This change in spatial orientation makes the hip on the side of the more adducted leg appear 'dysplastic', with shortening of the lower limb and asymmetry of the thigh skin creases.

The asymmetry may be more widespread owing to a generalized 'skeletal skew' involving the shape of the skull (plagiocephaly), the posture of the neck (torticollis), the spine (commonly a left thoracolumbar scoliosis), the thorax (with a rib hump and contralateral anterior chest prominence), the pelvis (which is rotated and tilted) and the inclination of the legs (Figs. 4.11–4.15). Apart from the effect that this has upon the hips, the leg lengths will appear unequal and the feet may seem to be 'windswept' (with calcaneovalgus of one and equinovarus or adduction of the other).

Differentiation of this transient, developmental condition from true displacement of the hip is often difficult (Weinberg & Pogrund 1980) and it may be that the two syndromes merge with each other. Clinical examination should

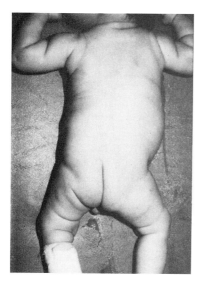
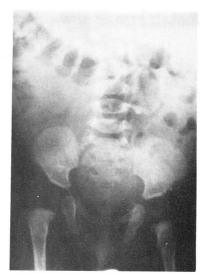

Fig. 4.11 A child with 'skeletal skew' causing the left hip to appear dysplastic. Note the associated right hip 'abductor contracture', the resultant pelvic obliquity and rotation, the right-sided lumbar scoliosis and the plaster splinting a mild left club foot deformity.

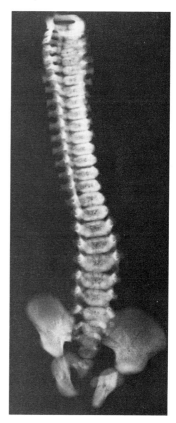

Fig. 4.12 The axial skeleton of an infant showing the skeletal skew.

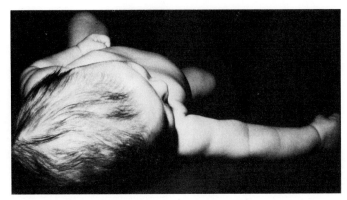

Fig. 4.13 A left plagiocephaly and thoracic moulding in the same child as shown in Fig. 4.11. The infant preferred to lie on his right side.

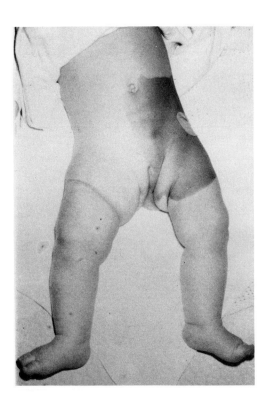

Fig. 4.14 A girl with a similar right hip abductor contracture and an apparent displacement of the left hip such that an arthrogram was felt to be advisable.

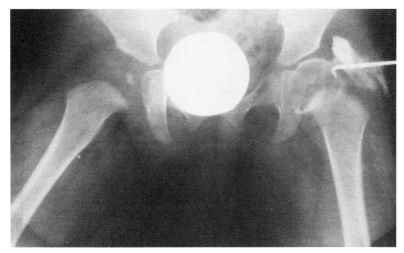

Fig. 4.15 The arthrogram shows a concentrically positioned left femoral head which was entirely stable clinically.

not only include an assessment of the hips with the infant lying supine, emphasizing in particular any limitation of abduction with the thighs flexed to 90°, but a review of the posture and hip movements with the baby prone. The hip opposite the adducted and spuriously dysplastic hip may present with an abductor contracture causing limited adduction (Figs. 4.16 and 4.17). This 'rotational dysplasia' (Catterall 1982) may represent an immaturity of positional reflexes and does not bear a close relationship with the fetal moulding noted at birth (Dunn 1976, Wilkinson 1985). The mother may remark upon the fact that her child prefers to lie on one side rather than the other, and in these cases the uppermost hip is the one that appears dysplastic. However there is no fixed relationship between the side of the suspicious hip and either the side of habit-lying or the pattern of the skeletal skew.

The self-limiting condition of skeletal and hip skewing should be recognized as benign because of the risks of abduction at this age (see later under 'pressure lesions of the proximal femur'). A wait-and-see policy is justifiable in most cases, with radiographic review at 3-monthly intervals. Pelvic films should be carefully orientated using the horizontal line provided either by Hilgenreiner's line or a line joining the tips of the ischial tuberosities (Fig. 4.18). Rotational artefacts are revealed by comparing the obturator foramina (Tönnis 1976) or the width of the iliac wings (Macnicol 1985). The acetabular index is very variable, reflecting the differing rates of pelvic ossification (Perkins 1928; Table 4.3). When there is doubt about the stability of the hip, videoarthrography offers a dynamic assessment of the articulation. The position of the labrum and the absence or presence of an inturned limbus can be portrayed (Figs. 4.19–4.23), while a push–pull manoeuvre demonstrates the resistance of the soft tissues to deformation. If there is any instability, the position of the leg that achieves maximum congruity of the joint can be determined, and then adopted during later splintage. An eccentric position

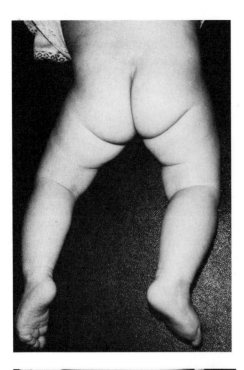

Fig. 4.16 A child with skeletal skew should be examined prone as well as supine. Note the abducted position of the left hip which was associated with apparently limited abduction of the right hip.

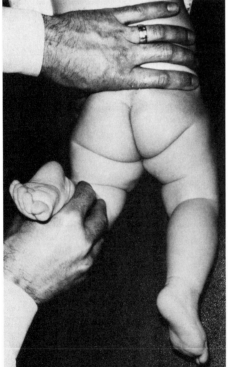

Fig. 4.17 The left hip abductor contracture prevents the leg from being adducted to the midline. Both hips were stable and presented with an equal range of total movement, although the arcs differed spatially. The condition resolved after the first year of life.

Fig. 4.18 The definition of hip dysplasia and displacement relies upon the ossification of the pelvis and femora and the lines that can be drawn at the edges of the iliac portion of the acetabulum. When assessing pelvic obliquity the line connecting the lowest points of the ischia is useful.

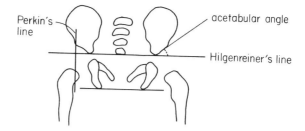

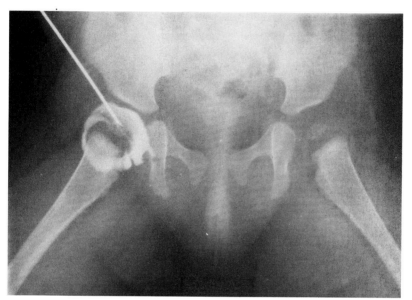

Fig. 4.19 The arthrogram shows that the labrum is deformed and there is medial pooling of dye, indicating that the femoral head is displaced.

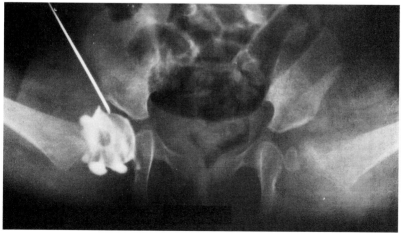

Fig. 4.20 After a month of abduction splintage the femoral head lies congruously below a normal labrum. The same appearance was present when the legs were positioned as in Fig. 4.19. Note the improved growth of the right acetabulum demonstrated by the previous growth arrest line.

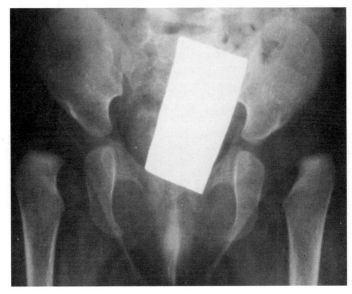

Fig. 4.21 A pelvic radiograph confirming bilateral dislocations of the hip in a six-month old infant.

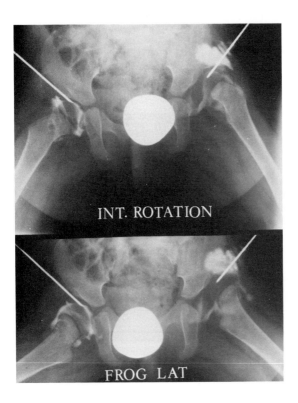

Fig. 4.22 After a period of skin traction the right hip could be reduced but the left hip remained dislocated until an arthrotomy enabled the obstructing capsule and labrum (the 'limbus') to be removed.

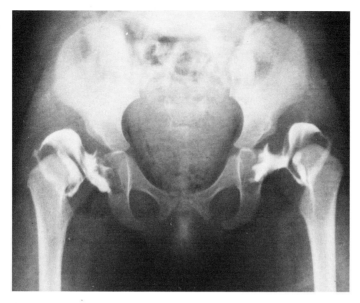

Fig. 4.23 Bilateral dislocations that were irreducible without surgery, on account of the soft tissue obstructions shown by arthrography.

Table 4.3 Radiographic features of the unstable hip in infancy. (The dysplastic changes that occur are open to considerable misinterpretation, particularly the slope of the acetabular roof or acetabular angle.)

'Putti's triad' (1933)
1. smaller or absent proximal femoral ossification centre
2. proximal femur placed laterally and high
3. sloping acetabular roof (increased inclination)

Table 4.4 Arthrographic features of hip displacement.

lateral (eccentric) position of femoral head		
medial pooling of contrast medium		
deformation of labrum:	I	no 'rosethorn' superiorly
	II	distortion of its concave inferior surface
	III	lateral edge lies above Hilgenreiner's line
	IV	no longer envelops femoral head.

Note The limbus represents an inturned fold of capsule and the deformed labrum (Fig. 4.23) and intrudes between the femoral head and the capsule posteriorly as well as superiorly.

of the femoral head secondary to an intra-articular obstruction (Fig. 4.24 and Table 4.4) then makes it necessary to decide upon open reduction immediately or nearer walking age (Mackenzie *et al.* 1960).

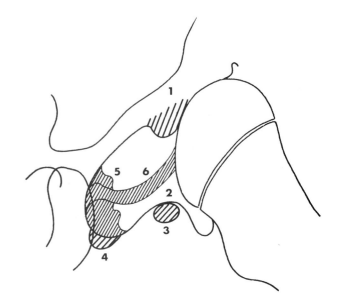

Fig. 4.24 Structures which may prevent reduction of the femoral head: (1) the limbus, (2) the inferior capsule of the hip joint, (3) the psoas tendon, (4) the transverse acetabular ligament, (5) the acetabular fat pad or pulvinar, (6) the ligamentum teres (if hypertrophied).

Treatment of the toddler (12–24 months)

Some of the children who present later than the first year may have been missed in spite of neonatal screening, and these false negative cases at birth may presumably be decreased in number by greater attention to screening procedures. This supposition has been questioned (Mackenzie & Wilson 1981, Wilkinson 1985) and it is impossible to resolve this issue, at least at present, because of the great disparity between the success of different, regional programmes. However, it is apparent that the child presenting with a displaced hip at a later age has a stronger family history of the condition (Wynne-Davies 1970b), and the abnormality manifests equally on the left or right sides in distinction to the left-sided predominance at birth.

Sadly, the clinical features of the dislocating hip are not appreciated as significant by the parents, or fail to be recognized by the family doctor, in approximately half the cases. A delay in diagnosis is therefore all too common during the second year of life, any asymmetry in gait being put down to habit. Bilateral hip displacement is even slower to be detected but clinical signs are usually unequivocal if the toddler is properly examined. In addition to the alterations in gait (Table 4.5), the following changes are present:

1 The physiognomy of the affected hip is altered with a high greater trochanter,

flattening of the buttock and a hollow below the femoral triangle (sign of Joachimsthal 1908).

2   A true shortening of the leg. Perkin's sign (1928), whereby the hips and knees are flexed with the child lying supine and the heights of the respective knees are compared, is accurate in the older child but may be difficult to gauge in the plump toddler with a subluxing hip.

3   A loss of total hip movements, not simply abduction, and therefore distinguishable from a case of skeletal skew; restriction of abduction, with the hip flexed to 90°, is an early sign of displacement and testing for this may produce discomfort (Table 4.5).

4   In the child with ligament laxity instability of the hip can sometimes be discerned.

Table 4.5 Presentation of hip dislocation in the toddler.

Delay in walking
Short leg with tip-toe walking
Limp (short leg and positive Trendelenburg types)
'Funny' walk
Dragging leg
Asymmetry (including drooping shoulder)
Externally rotated leg
Abnormal shoe wear
(Previous difficulty in crawling)

Asymmetry of the thigh skin creases is open to misinterpretation but may be obvious in a toddler with unilateral hip dislocation. In bilateral cases the abnormalities may be difficult to detect since they are symmetrical, but the waddling gait is characteristic, while the proximal migration of the greater trochanters gives the pelvis a female rather than male appearance. Associated orthopaedic conditions should also be sought, including generalized ligament laxity, the stigmata of myelodysplasia with particular reference to calf girths and foot deformities, and metabolic disease or dysplasias affecting the rest of the skeleton.

Displacement of the hip has now advanced though several stages and becomes progressively more difficult to reverse:

neonatal hip → mild displacement → subluxation → dislocation (or
instability   on provocation   acetabular
('primary   ('preluxation')   dysplasia with a
dysplasia')   subluxated femoral
                                                           head)

The precise change in the morphology of the soft tissues of the hip joint varies from case to case, as will the way in which they obstruct the femoral head from entering the introitus (Fig. 4.24). Some femoral heads dislocate completely and rest within a false acetabulum whereas others remain subluxed and therefore in apposition with the upper margin of the true acetabulum. In the latter case the prognosis following surgical reduction may be worse since deformation of the acetabulum as well as the femoral head occurs with the passage of time.

Decisions about the nature of the soft tissue obstructions are immeasurably improved by arthrography after a few weeks of skin traction. Le Veuf (1947) reported the arthrographic appearance of the hip in a careful study before and after reduction of the femoral head. Irregularities and filling defects are readily demonstrated

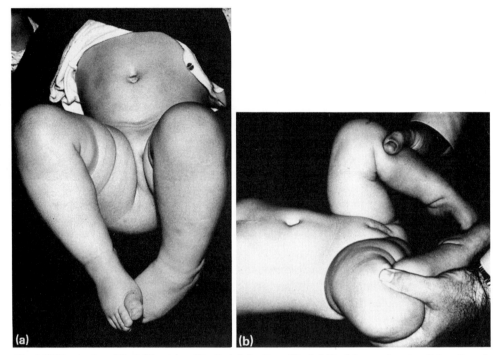

Fig. 4.25 Shortening of the left leg (a) and limited abduction of the left hip (b) secondary to a dislocation of the femoral head.

Table 4.6 Indications for open reduction.

irreducible dislocation
unstable reduction (requiring extreme positioning of the leg)
eccentric 'reduction' (indicating an incarcerated soft tissue obstruction)
redislocation

'The quality of reduction dominates the outcome . . . ' *George C. Lloyd Roberts (in Tachdjian 1982)*
'No complete or permanent restoration of function occurs without a perfect anatomical restoration'
Putti (1933)

(Mitchell 1963) and any evidence of eccentricity when the femoral head is resting in the concavity of the acetabulum indicates that open reduction is advisable (Wilkinson 1985). The rate of surgical exploration inevitably increases with the age of the child (Table 4.6) while the likelihood of establishing a concentric reduction correspondingly decreases since deformities of the femoral head and alteration in the shape of the acetabulum gradually develop.

Videoarthrography once more offers a dynamic portrayal of the soft tissue obstacles to reduction, and the most suitable position of the leg for the maintenance of congruent reduction. Flexion and abduction (the Lorenz position) is preferable to extension and internal rotation (the Lange position) since the latter will accentuate the degree of femoral anteversion. The position of the femoral head and the orientation of the acetabulum can also be assessed by the following investigations:

1   lateral, ('cross table') views (Chuinard 1978), although their interpretation is often difficult;
2   stereophotogrammetry (Weintroub *et al.* 1981) which is a complex measurement derived from specific radiographic views;
3   computerized axial tomography (Figs. 4.26 & 4.27) which is of value when the bones have ossified but exposes the child to appreciable X-irradiation and loses precision if a metal implant is present;
4   magnetic resonance, which reveals the soft tissues well and has a greater application than axial tomography.

Closed versus open reduction

Reduction of the femoral head must never be forced, and should be preceded by a period of skin traction and an arthrogram after the age of 3 months. The femoral head is easily deformed during the first year of life and its resistance to injury is proportional to the degree of ossification. Therefore any obstruction to gentle reduction should either be removed surgically, or attempts at relocating the femoral head should be delayed until the child is approximately one year of age (Somerville & Scott 1957).

Longitudinal traction with the infant in a slightly head-down position is satisfactory under the age of six months, although no more than a week of such treatment is advised. After this age, gallows traction (Figs 4.28 & 4.29) is effective and allows the toddler great freedom of movement while the secondary muscle contractures are being stretched. However, ischaemic changes in the feet may occur after the age of three years, particularly if the knees are held extended. Frame reduction (Scott 1953, Mitchell 1985) is an alternative method of applying traction, this time with the hips extended. Once the femoral head has been brought down to the acetabulum the legs are gradually abducted and a cross-pull can be applied in the more difficult case (Fig. 4.30). However, the frame demands nursing care of a standard that is not always available and its use is now limited.

Adductor tenotomy may be required but it is difficult to support the contention that it is always necessary (Mackenzie *et al.* 1960). The time that skin traction is applied depends upon the age of the child, and in the case of frame reduction, upon the appearances of serial radiographs obtained at weekly intervals. How far

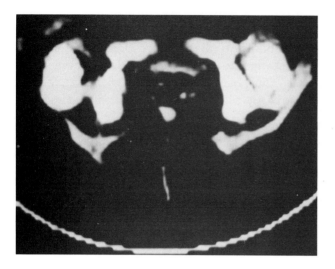

Fig. 4.26 A CT scan (computerized axial tomography) showing a posteriorly dislocated left hip.

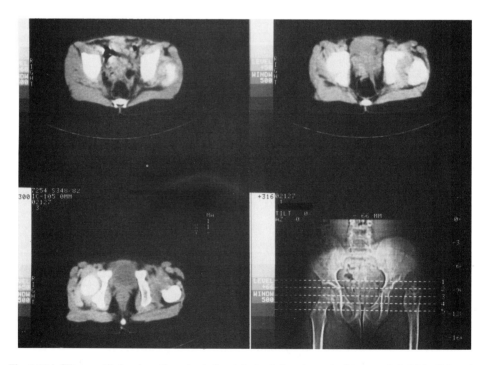

Fig. 4.27 A CT scan will also show the extent of acetabular deformity, as in this case of a left hip dislocation secondary to septic arthritis.

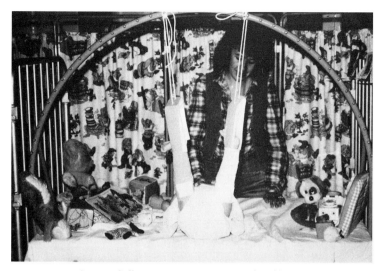

Fig. 4.28 Gallows traction using an overhead hoop.

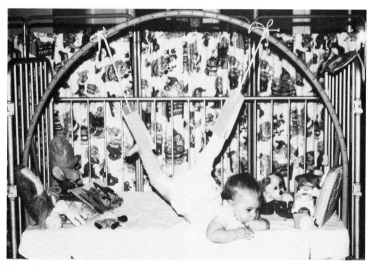

Fig. 4.29 The child is free to move about since the only intention is that the soft tissues around the hip should be stretched.

the legs should be abducted is uncertain. Hoop traction readily achieves 45° of abduction but Wilkinson (1985) considers that the postreduction range of abduction may be restricted if a greater range is not obtained at the traction stage. Reduction on a frame regularly produces 90° of hip abduction, although this requires approximately six weeks of treatment before surgery. If difficulties arise it is preferable to consider a femoral shortening with open reduction of the femoral head, rather than to resort to skeletal traction and weights in excess of two kilograms.

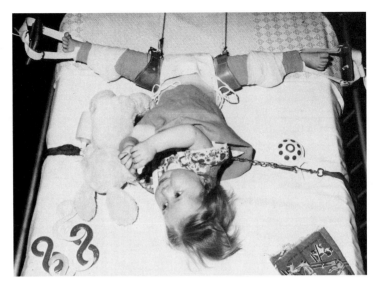

Fig. 4.30 Cross pull may help to lower the femoral heads when full abduction has been achieved, with or without the abduction frame.

If closed manipulation results in a congruous reduction arthrographically the leg is splinted in a plaster spica (Fig. 4.31) using a modified Lorenz position of 90° of flexion and up to 60° of abduction. The precise position that ensures maximum congruity is maintained during the application of the spica using an adjustable plaster table (Fig. 4.32). The plaster should be carefully moulded over the posterior and lateral prominences of the greater trochanter, and should initially include the knee in order to control rotation of the femur. After one month the spica is changed under a general anaesthetic which allows the stability of the hip to be reassessed manually and radiographically. The second plaster can be abbreviated if the hip feels stable (Fig. 4.33) and the hips can be 'deflexed' to just under 90°, with abduction of approximately 45°. By the end of the second month it is often possible to apply an abduction brace (Fig. 4.34) instead of a spica, although this decision is influenced by the growth response of the acetabulum.

After the age of three years the capacity of the acetabulum to respond tails off markedly, partly because of decreasing biological plasticity and partly because of the progressive difficulty in attaining a concentric reduction owing to the differential growth and gradual deformation of both the acetabulum and the dislocated femoral head. In a proportion of cases acetabular growth improves the depth and shape of the cup after the age of four years (Ponseti 1978, Weintroub *et al.* 1979) but it is virtually impossible to predict the acetabular response in each case, even if age is taken into consideration (Kasser *et al.* 1985).

The abduction brace or a Denis Browne harness controls the femoral position sufficiently to encourage further acetabular development (Smith *et al.* 1968, Lindstrom & Ponseti 1979) although these devices are poorly tolerated as the child grows larger. Pelvic osteotomy is to be preferred to a protracted period of splintage, particularly if the acetabular response is meagre.

A trial of closed reduction (Vickers & Catterall 1980) may produce acceptable results in the very young toddler where the soft tissue obstruction is more pliant. But the uncertainty of producing a stable and concentric reduction after the age of 18 months, and the reported avascular necrosis rate of 20%, seriously limit the value of this approach. An eccentric reduction cannot be accepted, and if the

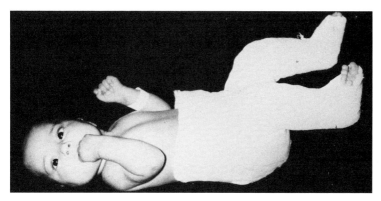

Fig. 4.31 A plaster spica controlling the postion of the femoral heads in an infant.

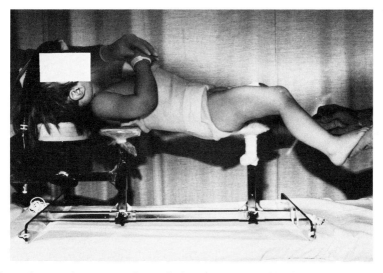

Fig. 4.32 The application of a spica is made simpler by using an adjustable plaster table. Note the supports under the sacrum, shoulders and head.

videoarthrogram shows the femoral head to remain displaced despite variations in the position of the leg, immediate open reduction is advised (Table 4.6). The soft tissue obstructions that are encountered (Fig. 4.24) are collectively or individually responsible for narrowing the introitus. The limbus need not be

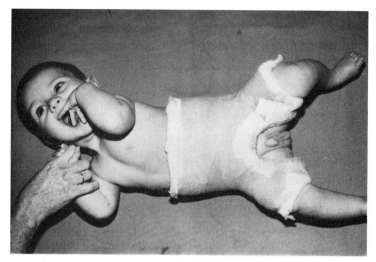

Fig. 4.33 An abbreviated ('pantaloon') spica of Baycast which permits active rotation of the thighs.

removed if it can still be hooked out of the socket and brought over the circumference of the femoral head. In the older child the limbus ceases to be so malleable although it can still be delivered over the femoral head in certain cases if radial cuts are made in the labrum in order to loosen it. Excision of the irreversibly deformed limbus has been recommended strongly by Somerville (1982), Mitchell (1983) and Wilkinson (1985). The procedure is possible through a small anterior approach or posteriorly and is followed by four weeks in a plaster spica and then a derotation varus proximal femoral osteotomy. An alternative approach is to carry out a more formal open reduction through either an anterolateral, posterior or medial (Ludloff 1913, Ferguson 1973) approach.

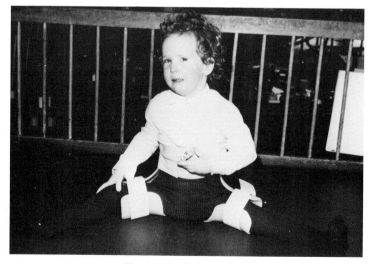

Fig. 4.34 An abduction brace.

The medial approach is ineffectual when a rigidly deformed limbus is present and may additionally endanger the vascularity of the femoral head. The Lorenz position is preferred to the Lange position after reduction since anteversion of the proximal femur is rarely gross, and cannot be deduced accurately from the range of internal rotation of the hip in a child who often has lax ligaments. Furthermore, anteversion tends to correct after concentric reduction of the hip, but may be increased if the femur is extended and forceably internally rotated.

Plaster splintage following open reduction is similar to that after closed reduction, although the time in a spica may be longer. An abduction brace is preferred to broomstick plasters unless it is felt necessary to control rotation as well as abduction. The radiographs following open reduction must be carefully monitored for any signs of redislocation since an immediate change of position in plaster, or a femoral osteotomy, then becomes necessary.

Pressure ('avascular') lesions of the proximal femur

It has already been noted in this chapter that the cartilaginous femoral head (Fig. 4.35) is very susceptible to injury as a result of both pressure of its contour against segments of the acetabulum or a soft tissue obstruction, and also forced positions

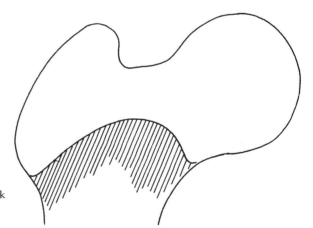

Fig. 4.35 The femoral head, neck and greater trochanter are fully cartilaginous in the neonate.

of the thigh, particularly abduction. In part the damage is incurred by the effects of unequal pressures upon growth of the head and neck, and in part by ischaemia. The changes in blood supply to the proximal femur at different ages are well known (Trueta 1957, Ogden 1974), and although some vessels may reach the femoral head from the neck despite the presence of the growth plate, vascularity is principally dependent upon the retinacular vessels in the hip joint capsule and the ligamentum teres. Fig. 4.36 shows the arteries that feed the capsular vessels and interruption of those vessels in relation to the trochanteric anastomosis or the retinacular fibres will endanger the epiphysis and growth plate.

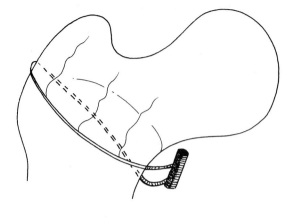

Fig. 4.36 The medial (posterior) and lateral (anterior) circumflex arteries supply the proximal femur from the profunda femoris artery.

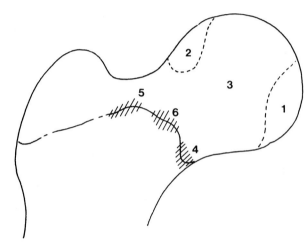

Fig. 4.37 Sites of pressure (ischaemic) lesions of the proximal femur. (1) medial epiphysial, (2) superior epiphysis, (3) total epiphysis, (4) medial growth plate, (5) lateral growth plate, (6) total growth plate.

Table 4.7 Pressure lesions (avascular necrosis) of the proximal femur.

Femoral head (epiphysis)	transient irregularity of ossification with possible coxa magna and incongruity later medial (1), causing a triangulate head superior (2), causing superior notching total (3), leading to coxa magna/plana and gross incongruity
Growth plate (physis)	medial (4), causing a varus femoral neck lateral (5), causing a short, valgus neck and an oval femoral head total (6), leading to a short, wide neck and variable head deformity.

Combined femoral head and growth plate lesion causing major deformity of the head and neck with incongruity.

In all pressure lesions there is a relative overgrowth of the greater trochanter and partial growth arrest of the superior rim of the acetabulum is common.

Note The numbers in brackets refer to the sites of the lesions as shown in Fig. 4.37.

The radiographic changes that follow pressure and ischaemia of the proximal femur have been described in a number of papers (Salter *et al.* 1969, Gage & Winter 1972, Bucholz & Ogden 1978, Kalamchi & MacEwen 1980, Bertol *et al.* 1982) with particular reference to the dangers of forced or rigid splintage of the hips in the infant, and the risks associated with inappropriate closed reduction. Although evidence in favour of a pre-reduction period of skin traction is not entirely convincing, there is no doubt that closed reduction is increasingly risky as the child grows older (Vickers & Catterall 1980), particularly if soft tissue contractures have not been lengthened by a period of traction. Open reduction, whereby the capsule, psoas tendon and adductor muscles can be sectioned, may be an acceptable solution in cases where traction has played little or no part in the initial management.

Table 4.7 outlines the various forms of injury sustained by the epiphysis and growth plate. The lesions may be partial or complete, and the major sites of involvement are shown in Fig. 4.37. The femoral head may show nothing more than a temporary irregularity of ossification, or may even escape injury in spite of significant inhibition of the growth plate (Fig. 4.38). Combined lesions (Fig. 4.39) distort not only the mechanics of the hip joint but also the articular surfaces such that major disability can be predicted. Prevention of these iatrogenic lesions is the only effective remedy.

Treatment of the young child (2–6 years)

In the preschool child every effort should be made to stabilize a hip that still shows signs of displacing. This requires regular clinical and radiographic review of all cases where development of the acetabulum gives cause for concern, or where femoral anteversion remains excessive. The combination of increased acetabular and femoral anteversion is always likely to produce a progressive subluxation, which will eventually become irreversible as the two surfaces of the joint become incongruent. Surgical correction of the acetabulum, the proximal femur or both components must be recommended before this deformation occurs.

The indications and timing of pelvic and femoral osteotomies vary greatly between surgeons of equivalent experience, and it is therefore invidious to suggest that only one method of management will suffice. Some form of redirectional acetabular procedure or acetabuloplasty will be required in approximately half the children discovered to have displacement of the hip at the early walking stage. Diagnosis at a later age results in an increasingly greater incidence of osteotomy, and in some children it will be necessary to carry out repeat osteotomies, let alone procedures on both sides of the joint.

Pelvic osteotomy

Only the more commonly described procedures will be discussed in this chapter, although the range of operations available for the dysplastic or subluxed hip is

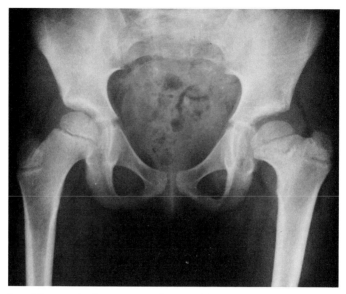

Fig. 4.38 A lesion of the growth plate causing a shortened femoral neck and relative overgrowth of the greater trochanter.

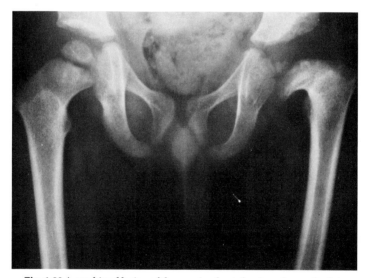

Fig. 4.39 A combined lesion of the proximal epiphysis and growth plate.

considerable. The innominate osteotomy of Salter (1961) is suitable for the child between the ages of two and six years with a dislocated hip, and is appropriate for the subluxing hip in the older child and adolescent. The hip should present with a virtually normal range of movement and should be reducible into the acetabulum before the osteotomy is done. It is difficult to be certain that a congruous reduction has been obtained at the initial exploration, and for this reason, as well as the fact that the soft tissues may be under some tension, a staged procedure may be advisable. Hence an open reduction and plaster fixation of the hip in the Lorenz position can be followed six weeks later with the innominate osteotomy, or a preliminary period in plasters and bracing may be tried in the child of 18–24 months before considering the osteotomy. Since the Salter procedure lengthens the affected leg it may be necessary to carry out an initial varus-rotation osteotomy (Morscher 1978). At a later age, when traction is contraindicated, the Salter procedure should be combined with femoral shortening (Klisić & Jankovic 1976). This releases tension in the flexors, extensors and adductors of the hip as long as the psoas and rectus femoris tendons are released separately. An abductor contracture is avoided by permitting the abductors to slide distally from the ridge of the iliac crest.

The technique of the Salter procedure is clearly described (Salter 1961) although a transverse, skin crease incision is now preferred to the iliofemoral approach. The steps in the operation described by Salter must be adhered to and it is particularly important to expose the capsule as fully as possible. Psoas tenotomy is required, as this tendon is a major deforming force, and is best achieved by rolling the tendon forwards with a blunt hook just above the lesser trochanter, well away from the femoral nerve. The initial dissection of the abductors should be taken at least to the zenith of the iliac wing, thus relaxing gluteus medius and minimus, and the adductors may be released percutaneously through a separate, small groin incision. In children with a dislocation the capsule must be opened and any obstruction removed as with an open reduction. In addition to the inturned limbus, the transverse acetabular ligament and inferior capsule may be obstructive (Howorth 1963), thus causing a diaphragm of tissue to extend across the acetabular rim. Medial structures, particularly the ligamentum teres and pulvinar (fat pad), are often hypertrophic but opinion is divided as to whether they should be excised. The ligamentum teres is a useful guide into the depths of the true acetabulum and should certainly be preserved until circumferential obstructing tissues have been removed. Even after extensive soft tissue dissection the femoral head may not seat as deeply in the acetabulum as desired, especially in the older child in whom a significant incongruity has developed between the femoral head and the acetabulum.

Figs. 4.40–4.42 show the site of the osteotomy and the bone graft in place. In order to move the distal fragment as far distally, anteriorly and laterally as possible the leg should be flexed over the opposite lower limb and the graft inserted with the head dislocated. However, subsequent replacement of the femoral head must ensure adequate reduction. The osteotomy should not be opened up posteromedially and it is advisable to pull down the distal fragment gently and in stages, using the flat of an osteotome in addition to the guiding effect of a towel clip inserted in the bone immediately above the acetabulum. The capsulorrhaphy is an important part of the operation and should tighten the lax capsule so that the position of the femoral head is controlled and the leg tends to lie in internal rotation.

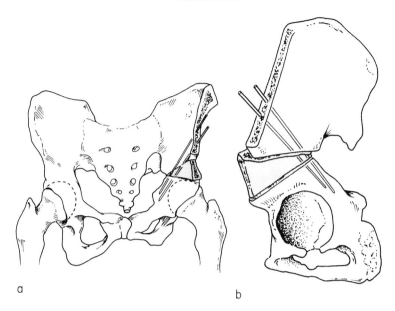

Fig. 4.40 The Salter innominate osteotomy (a) anteroposterior view, (b) lateral view.

The graft is secured with two stout Kirschner wires, preferably threaded, and these should not be cut too short as they are removed subsequently. A one and one half hip spica is used to splint the leg in slight flexion, abduction and internal rotation for six weeks.

Complications may occur with the innominate osteotomy, particularly redislocation of the femoral head which may be either posterior or anterior. Also reported are slippage or absorption of the bone graft, acetabular penetration by the wires, injury to the sciatic nerve or superior gluteal artery, and distortion of the iliac wing. Local wound problems such as haematoma, infection and damage to the lateral femoral cutaneous nerve are relatively uncommon.

Femoral osteotomy

Corrective osteotomy of the proximal femur is an established procedure either in its own right or as an adjunct to a previous pelvic osteotomy. If the osteotomy is to be used as a primary operation, the subsequent acetabular development must be carefully monitored and an acetabular realignment or acetabuloplasty carried out if the appearances suggest inadequate femoral head cover. Rotation femoral osteotomy, whereby the distal fragment is rotated externally, will both correct excessive anteversion of the femur and tighten the capsule of the joint by a screw-home mechanism. A break in Shenton's arc is therefore corrected, and this effect may be checked preoperatively by an internal rotation radiographic view of the hip. The introduction of 10–15° of varus with the rotation is advisable as this corrects the commonly associated valgus deformity of the proximal femur and anticipates

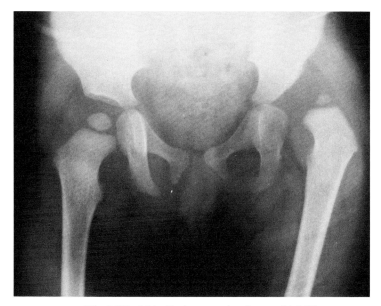

Fig. 4.41 Left hip displacement in a 2-year-old child.

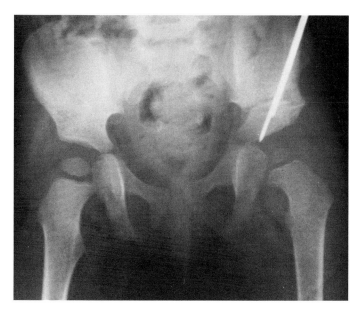

Fig. 4.42 The radiographic appearance after a Salter osteotomy. Further lateral acetabular growth can be anticipated.

the femoral overgrowth which occurs subsequent to the osteotomy (Mitchell 1985).

The therapeutic effects of varus rotation femoral osteotomy are maximal before the age of 4 years, but after the age of 8 years the osteotomy has little or no influence upon acetabular development although it may still redistribute beneficially the mechanical loading of the hip joint (Kasser *et al.* 1985). The inclusion of 10–20° of extension at the osteotomy site may also be indicated (Catterall 1982) and repeated femoral osteotomies may be required over a period of approximately six years. However, the need for several femoral procedures is always a worrying feature and may indicate a persistent malalignment of the acetabulum, incongruent reduction of the femoral head or a significant neuromuscular imbalance. The inconsistent response of the hip to varus rotation osteotomy (Gibson & Benson 1982) therefore suggests that it is better utilized as a secondary procedure to innominate osteotomy, and that the best time to resort to these osteotomies is before the age of 4 years. After that age the outcome after either pelvic or femoral osteotomy is progressively more uncertain, even if a femoral shortening and combined osteotomies (Klisić & Jankovic 1976) are attempted (Figs. 4.43 & 4.44).

Osteotomy of the proximal femur is readily carried out through a lateral thigh incision at the intertrochanteric region. In the toddler or young child the shaft is

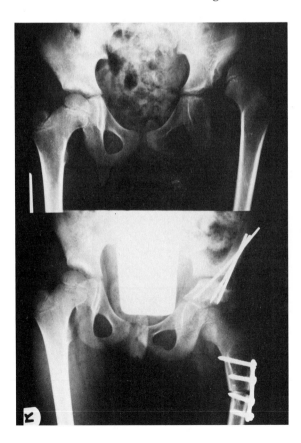

Fig. 4.43 A left hip dislocation treated by femoral shortening and a Salter osteotomy. The lower picture was taken 2 months later.

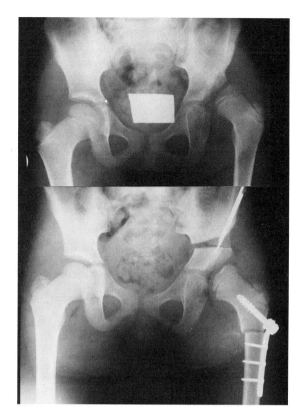

Fig. 4.44 A left hip subluxation treated by femoral shortening and a Salter osteotomy. The lower picture was taken one month later.

cut subperiosteally and fixation in the corrected position secured initially with a number 8 four-hole Sherman plate prebent to give 15° of varus (Mitchell 1983). The distal fragment is externally rotated until only 10° of internal rotation is possible with the hip extended, and the plate is applied to the lateral surface of the femur. If some extension is required at the osteotomy it may be easier to apply the plate over the anterior surface of the bone. A plaster spica splints the leg in the corrected position for six weeks, following which physiotherapy is started. In the older child fixation is possible with the Coventry screw and plate or a blade-plate device. The Richard's juvenile implant may not provide sufficient antirotational support for the proximal fragment, and plaster spica support is advised for all children up to the age of six years.

Treatment after early childhood

The orthopaedic management of congenital dislocation or dysplasia of the hip becomes progressively more unsatisfactory the older the child is at presentation. In a proportion of children, previous conservative or operative treatment may have failed to secure a congruous reduction, or acetabular development may have remained inadequate. The features of acetabular dysplasia are listed in Table 4.8.

Table 4.8 Clinical presentation of acetabular dysplasia.

Groin pain (initially from capsular tension and therefore present during exertion rather than rest)
Referred pain (knee, proximal thigh, trochanteric region, buttock)
Limp (Trendelenburg — with positive delayed, and then immediate, Trendelenburg test 1895)
Long or short leg
Anterior lump sign (Fig. 4.45)
Wasting of buttock or thigh
Limited hip movements (loss of abduction, flexion, flexion-adduction and rotation)
Clunking or clicking in the hip
Generalized ligament laxity

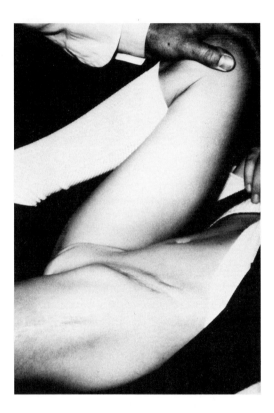

Fig. 4.45 An anterior 'lump sign' augmented by flexing the opposite hip.

It is rare to encounter dysplasia of the acetabulum without some deformity of the femoral head, but it is important to distinguish between a joint that is still biomechanically stable and one that is irreversibly subluxed. In the former case, a reconstructive pelvic osteotomy is still possible (Fig. 4.42) whereas in the subluxated hip a salvage procedure such as the Chiari pelvic osteotomy is indicated (Mitchell 1974). When a lump sign is present (Fig. 4.45) irreversible deformation of the hip joint has occurred, making the surgical construction of a congruent hip impossible.

Pain is experienced as the weight of the child increases, and usually becomes persistent during adolescence or in early adult life. The disability that is experienced can be graded (Table 4.9) and is the product of inadequate femoral head cover and shearing forces between the femoral head and the acetabulum. Pain probably arises from the stretching of the capsule and protective muscle spasm in the early stages. Later, the inflammatory process of osteoarthritis is responsible for the symptoms at rest and the increasing degree of stiffness in the hip. Conservative measures such as rest, weight loss, leg length equalization by means of a contralateral shoe raise and physiotherapy are unlikely to be effective for long, and some form of surgical treatment is indicated in order to retard the degeneration of the joint.

Table 4.9 Gradation of hip disability.

Grade 1	Painless hip with normal function
Grade 2	Occasional ache and limp with normal walking speed but more fatigue
Grade 3	Intermittent pain with persistent slight limp and reduced walking speed and endurance
Grade 4	Persistent pain and obvious limp with further restriction of function
Grade 5	Severe pain even at rest with grossly reduced walking speed and distance

Although the treatment of hip dysplasia during adolescence cannot be discussed in detail, principles of surgical management can be outlined.

1   If there is a symptomatic, persistent femoral anteversion, this can be satisfactorily corrected by means of a proximal femoral osteotomy using a blade-plate (Figs. 4.46–4.48). Correction of femoral alignment alone will suffice if acetabular development is reasonably normal (Severin 1941, grades I and II; Table 4.10).

2   A coexistent 'long leg dysplasia' can be treated with a varus component to the osteotomy, and further shortening can be produced by removing a segment of the proximal femur.

3   When the acetabulum affords poor femoral head cover but the joint remains reasonably congruous and stable (Severin grade III) a redirectional osteotomy of the acetabulum is required (Salter 1961, Eppwright 1975, Sutherland & Greenfield 1977, Steel 1977, Wagner 1978, Ninomiya & Tagawa 1984). Many other variations of this osteotomy have been described but the principle remains the same, namely, to bring the articular cartilage of the acetabulum over the dome of the femoral head (Fig. 4.49). Acetabuloplasty (Pemberton 1958, Marafioti & Westin 1980) is no longer possible at this age, and none of these osteotomies address the problem of insufficient acetabular volume.

4   For Severin grades IV and V the Chiari medial displacement osteotomy is an appropriate method of buttressing the femoral head (Macnicol *et al.* 1981) without making any attempt to reduce the subluxated or dislocated femoral head (Fig. 4.50). Wagner (1978) has described a combined procedure (the type III spherical osteotomy) in which the acetabulum is both rotated and buttressed by a modified Chiari procedure.

5   As with pelvic osteotomy at an earlier age, it may be necessary to carry out an additional proximal femoral osteotomy, ensuring varus, valgus (Ninomiya & Tagawa 1984), rotation or extension, depending upon the position of the femur which secures maximum congruency of the joint.

6   Other forms of proximal femoral or acetabular surgery (Table 4.11) have a minor part to play in the management of late displacement of the hip.

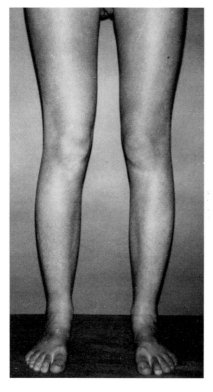

Fig. 4.46 Femoral anteversion causes the knees to point medially.

Table 4.10 Grading of hip dysplasia (after Severin 1941).

Grade 1	Normal articulation with a congruous, spherical femoral head and an acetabulum providing at least 90% cover (CE angle* over 25° in adults or over 15° between the ages of 6 and 14 years.
Grade 2	A stable hip but with possible mild coxa magna and reduced acetabular cover such that the CE angle is between 20° and 25°.
Grade 3	Femoral head deformity sufficient to produce mild incongruity but without obvious subluxation despite further reduction in the CE angle (10–20° in the adult and under 15° in the child).
Grade 4	Inadequate femoral head cover allowing irreversible displacement (subluxated head, Mitchell 1983). Shenton's line cannot be restored by internally rotating and abducting the leg; the CE angle becomes negative and incongruity is significant.
Grade 5	The femoral head is dislocated and resides in a secondary acetabulum. Acetabular dysplasia is severe.
Grade 6	Redislocation of the femoral head.

*Wiberg (1939)

The Chiari pelvic osteotomy is not advised before maturity, although it does stabilize effectively the hip in children with neurological conditions. The advantages, disadvantages and complications of the procedure are shown in Table 4.12 and the increased cover afforded the femoral head is clear in Fig. 4.50. Anterior cover is often deficient even after the osteotomy and therefore the use of a bone

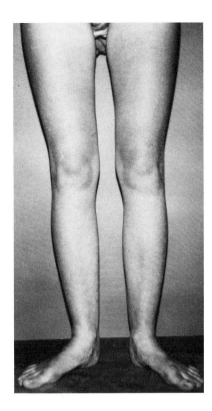

Fig. 4.47 When the knees face forwards a compensatory external tibial torsion is revealed.

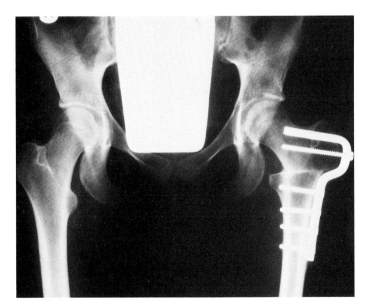

Fig. 4.48 Proximal femoral 'derotation' osteotomy with an AO blade plate has improved congruity of the left hip and reconstituted Shenton's line which was previously broken.

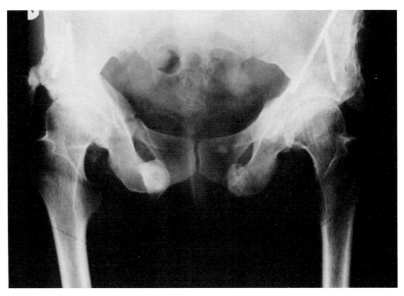

Fig. 4.49 The Steel triple osteotomy (1977) which realigns the acetabulum after transecting the innominate bone and the pubic and ischial rami.

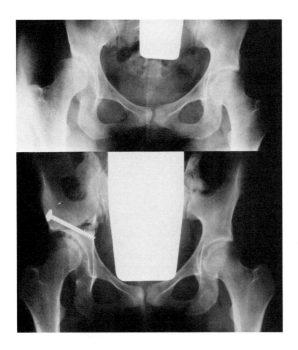

Fig. 4.50 Radiographic appearance before (above) and after (below) the medial displacement pelvic osteotomy of Chiari (1955).

graft from the iliac wing or a limited shelf procedure may enhance the therapeutic benefits of the osteotomy. Remarkable remodelling of the ilium occurs above the femoral head, which is protected in turn by the thickened capsule of the joint.

Table 4.11 Surgical options in the treatment of persistent acetabular incompetence.

1	Realignment pelvic osteotomy	Salter procedure (1961)
		Periacetabular procedures
		Eppwright (1975)
		Sutherland & Greenfield (1977)
		Steel (1977)
		Wagner (1978)
		Ninomiya & Tagawa (1984)
2	Acetabuloplasty	Pemberton (1958)
		'Pembersal' (Perlic *et al.* 1985)
3	Shelf procedure	König (1891)
		Hey-Groves (1927)
		Wilson (1974)
		Wainwright (1976)
4	Medial displacement pelvic osteotomy	Chiari (1955)
		Mitchell (1974)
5	Proximal femoral osteotomy	Varus-rotation
		Somerville (1982)
		Mitchell (1983)
		Kasser, Bowen & McEwen (1985)
		shortening Klisić & Jankovic (1976)
		valgus Ninomiya & Tagawa (1984)
		Lorenz 'bifurcation', Coleman (1978)
		Shanz 'pelvic-support', Coleman (1978)
6	Colonna (1947) procedure or Girdlestone arthroplasty	Coleman (1978)
7	Total hip prosthetic replacement	
8	Arthrodesis	

Note When the hip is reducible, 1, 2 & 5 are appropriate; shelf procedures (3) are less durable. When the hip is irreducible, 3, 4, 6, 7 and 8 are applicable as salvage procedures.

Table 4.12 Chiari pelvic osteotomy.

Advantages	femoral head decompression
	(a) increases surface contact of weightbearing head
	(b) acetabulum is not moved distally
	reliable stabilization of hip pivot
	extra-articular procedure with less risk of stiffening
Disadvantages	steepened true acetabulum (increases aclivity)
	potential risk of stress risers
	pelvic outlet narrowed
	acetabular growth adversely affected in childhood
Complications	intra-articular damage if osteotomy placed too low
	overdisplacement causing medial prolapse of hip
	sciatic nerve injury
	obstruction of pelvic outlet possible after bilateral osteotomies
	nonunion

Conclusion

The treatment of congenital displacement of the hip is most effective in the neonate. Throughout the stages of childhood, reduction is possible by careful attention to detail and a progressive reliance upon surgical procedures. The management of this condition thus requires experience and operative skills which are difficult to maintain if the clinical problem is not being faced regularly. There is therefore a case for regional centres dealing with dysplasia and dislocation of the hip, partly on account of the size of population that is needed to generate sufficient orthopaedic experience of the problem, and also because of the medicolegal consequences of missed or poorly treated cases. Screening is the most effective method of identifying the condition since hip displacement remains asymptomatic until later childhood, and the infant should be examined on several occasions during the first year of life as well as at birth.

An anatomically perfect reduction of the femoral head is vital to the success of any programme of treatment and the surgeon must be constantly alert to the dangers of pressure necrosis of the proximal femur and redisplacement of the hip. Irrevocable changes occur in the older child, such that the results of surgery become less predictable. In high, bilateral dislocations it may therefore be preferable to leave the child untreated, and the range of operations available to the orthopaedic surgeon (Table 4.11) indicates that no one way is necessarily best, nor that a normal hip will result from even the most carefully rendered surgery.

References

Andrén L. (1961) Aetiology and diagnosis of congenital dislocation of the hip in newborns. *Radiologie (Berlin)*, **1**, 89.

Andrén L. (1962) Pelvic instability in newborns. *Acta Radiologica*, [Suppl.] 212.

Bado J. L. (1963) Le deviazioni dalla normal nella embriogenesi del musculo e nella patogenesi di alcune malformazioni congenite. *Archivio 'Putti' di Chirurgie degli organi dimovimento*, **18**, 37.

Barlow T. G. (1962) Early diagnosis and treatment of congenital dislocation of the hip. *Journal of Bone and Joint Surgery*, **44B**, 292.

Bennet G. C., Catford J. & Wilkinson J. A. (1982) The incidence of, and results of screening for, congenital dislocation of the hip. *Journal of Bone and Joint Surgery*, **64B**, 176.

Bertol P., Macnicol M. F. & Mitchell G. P. (1982) Radiographic features of neonatal congenital dislocation of the hip joint. *Journal of Bone and Joint Surgery*, **64B**, 176.

Bucholz R. W. & Ogden J. A. (1978) Patterns of ischemic necrosis of the proximal femur — non-operatively treated congenital hip disease. In *The Hip: Proceedings of the Sixth Open Scientific Meeting of the Hip Society*, pp. 43–63 C. V. Mosby Co., Saint Louis.

Carter C. O. & Wilkinson J. A. (1964) Genetic and environmental factors in the aetiology of congenital dislocation of the hip. *Clinical Orthopaedics*, **33**, 119.

Catford J. C., Bennet G. C. & Wilkinson J. A. (1982) Congenital hip dislocation: an increasing and still uncontrolled disability. *British Medical Journal*, **11**, 1527–30.

Catterall A. (1982) Acetabular dysplasia. In Tachdjian M.O. (ed) *Congenital Dislocation of the Hip*, pp. 479–500. Churchill Livingstone, New York, Edinburgh, London and Melbourne.

Chiari K. (1955) Ergebnisse mit der Beckenosteotomie als Pfannendachplastik. *Zeitschrift Orthopedica*, **87**, 14–18.

Chuinard E. G. (1978) Lateral roentgenography in the diagnosis and treatment of dysplasia/dislocation of the hip. *Orthopaedics,* **1,** 130.

Clark N. M. P., Harcke H. T., McHugh P., Soo Lee M., Borns P. F. & MacEwen G. D. (1985) Real-time ultrasound in the diagnosis of congenital dislocation and dysplasia of the hip. *Journal of Bone and Joint Surgery,* **67B,** 406–12.

Coleman S. S. (1978) *Congenital Dysplasia and Dislocation of the Hip.* C. V. Mosby Company, St Louis.

Colonna P. C. (1947) Arthroplasty of the hip for congenital dislocation in children. *Journal of Bone and Joint Surgery,* **29,** 711.

Dunn P. M. (1976) Perinatal observations on the aetiology of congenital dislocation of the hip. *Clinical Orthopaedics,* **119,** 11–21.

Dunn P. M., Evans R. E., Thearle M. J., Griffiths H. E. D. & Witherow P. J. (1985) Congenital dislocation of the hip: early and late diagnosis and management compared. *Archives of Disease in Childhood,* **60,** 407–14.

Eppwright R. H. (1975) Dial osteotomy of the acetabulum in the treatment of dysplasia of the hip. *Journal of Bone and Joint Surgery,* **57A,** 1172.

Ferguson A. B. Jr. (1973) Primary open reduction of congenital dislocation of the hip using a medial adductor approach. *Journal of Bone and Joint Surgery,* **55A,** 671.

Fredensborg N. (1977) The results of early treatment of typical congenital dislocation of the hip in Malmo. *Journal of Bone and Joint Surgery,* **58B,** 272–6.

Gage J. R. & Winter R. B. (1972) Avascular necrosis of the capital femoral epiphysis as a complication of closed reduction of congenital dislocation of the hip. *Journal of Bone and Joint Surgery,* **54A,** 373.

Gibson P. H. & Benson M. K. D. (1982) Congenital dislocation of the hip. Review at maturity of 147 hips treated by excision of the limbus and derotation osteotomy. *Journal of Bone and Joint Surgery,* **64B,** 169–75.

Hey-Groves E. W. (1927) Some contributions to the reconstructive surgery of the hip. *British Journal of Surgery,* **14,** 486.

Howorth M. B. (1963) The etiology of congenital dislocation of the hip. *Clinical Orthopaedics,* **29,** 164–70.

Joachimsthal G. (1908) Die angeborene Hüftverenkung als Teilerscheinung anderer angeborener Anomalien. *Zeitschrift Orthopaedica Chirurgica,* **22,** 31.

Kalamchi A. & MacEwen G. D. (1980) Avascular necrosis following treatment of congenital dislocation of the hip. *Journal of Bone and Joint Surgery,* **62A,** 876.

Kasser J., Bowen J. R. & MacEwen G. D. (1985) Varus derotation osteotomy in the treatment of persistent dysplasia in congenital dislocation of the hip. *Journal of Bone and Joint Surgery,* **67A,** 195–202.

Klisić P. & Jankovic L. (1976) Combined procedure of open reduction and shortening of the femur in treatment of congenital dislocation of the hips in older children. *Clinical Orthopaedics,* **119,** 60.

König F. (1891) Osteoplastische Behandlung der Kongenitalen Hüftgelenksluxation (mit Demonstration eines Praparates). *Verhandlungen der Deutschen Gesselschaft für Chirurgie,* **20,** 75.

Le Damany P. (1912) *La Luxation Congenitale de la Hanche. Etudes d'Anatomie Comparée d'Anthropogenie Normale et Pathologique, Deductions Therapeutique.* Felix Alcan, Paris.

Le Veuf J. (1947) Primary congenital subluxation of the hip. *Journal of Bone and Joint Surgery,* **29,** 149–62.

Lindstrom J. R. & Ponseti I. V. (1979) Acetabular development after reduction in congenital dislocation of the hip. *Journal of Bone and Joint Surgery,* **61A,** 112–8.

Lloyd Roberts G. C. & Ratliff A. H. C. (1978) *Hip Disorders in Children.* Butterworth, London.

Ludloff K. (1913) The open reduction of the congenital hip dislocation by an anterior incision. *American Journal of Orthopedic Surgery,* **10,** 438–54.

Mackenzie I. G. & Wilson J. G. (1981) Problems encountered in the early diagnosis and management of congenital dislocation of the hip. *Journal of Bone and Joint Surgery,* **63B,** 38.

Mackenzie I. G., Seddon H. & Trevor D. (1960) Congenital dislocation of the hip. *Journal of Bone and Joint Surgery,* **62B,** 689.

Macnicol M. F., Uprichard H. & Mitchell G. P. (1981) Exercise testing after the Chiari pelvic osteotomy. *Journal of Bone and Joint Surgery,* **63B,** 48.

Macnicol M. F. (1985) Congenital dislocation of the hip: the value of radiography and neonatal screening. *Journal of Bone and Joint Surgery,* **67B,** 487.

Marafioti R. I. & Westin G. W. (1980) Factors influencing the results of acetabuloplasty in children. *Journal of Bone and Joint Surgery,* **62A,** 765.

Marx V. O. (1938) New observations in congenital dislocation of the hip in the newborn. *Journal of Bone and Joint Surgery,* **20,** 1095.

Mitchell G. P. (1963) Arthrography in congenital displacement of the hip. *Journal of Bone and Joint Surgery,* **45B,** 88–95.

Mitchell G. P. (1972) Problems in the early diagnosis and management of congenital dislocation of the hip. *Journal of Bone and Joint Surgery,* **54B,** 4.

Mitchell G. P. (1974) Chiari medial displacement osteotomy. *Clinical Orthopaedics,* **98,** 146.

Mitchell G. P. (1983) In *The Hip: Congenital Dislocation* Harris N. H. (ed) *Postgraduate Textbook of Clinical Orthopaedics,* pp. 96–109. Wright, Bristol, London, Boston.

Monticelli G. & Milella P. P. (1982) Indications for treatment of congenital dislocation of the hip by the surgical medial approach. In Tachdjian M. O. (ed) *Congenital Dislocation of the Hip,* pp. 385–400. Churchill Livingstone, New York, Edinburgh, London and Melbourne.

Morscher E. (1978) Our experience with Salter's innominate osteotomy in the treatment of hip dysplasia. In Weil U. H. (ed) *Progress in Orthopaedic Surgery,* **2,** p. 107. Springer-Verlag, Berlin.

Ninomiya S. & Tagawa H. (1984) Rotational acetabular osteotomy for the dysplastic acetabulum. *Journal of Bone and Joint Surgery,* **66A,** 430–6.

Ogden J. A. (1974) Changing patterns of proximal femoral vascularity. *Journal of Bone and Joint Surgery,* **56A,** 941.

Ortolani M. (1948) La lussazione congenita dell'anca: Nuovi criteri diagnostici e profilattico-correttivi. Cappelli, Bologna.

Palmén K. (1961) Preluxation of the hip joint: diagnosis and treatment in the newborn and the diagnosis of the hip joint in Sweden during the years 1948–1960. *Acta Paediatrica,* [Suppl] **129,** 50.

Palmén K. (1984) Prevention of congenital dislocation of the hip. *Acta Orthopaedica Scandinavica,* [Suppl] **55,** 208.

Pavlik A. (1957) Die funktionelle Behandlungs methode mittels Riemenbugel als Prinzip der Konservativen Therapie bei angeborenen Hüftgelenksverren kungen der Sauglinge. *Zeitschrift Orthopaedica,* **89,** 341.

Pemberton P. A. (1958) Osteotomy of the ilium with rotation of the acetabular roof for congenital dislocation of the hip. *Journal of Bone and Joint Surgery,* **40A,** 724.

Perkins G. Signs by which to diagnose congenital dislocation of the hip. *Lancet,* **1,** 648.

Perlic P. C., Westin W. & Marafioti R. L. (1985) A combination pelvic osteotomy for acetabular dysplasia in children. *Journal of Bone and Joint Surgery,* **67A,** 842–50.

Ponseti I. V. (1978) Growth and development of the acetabulum in the normal child. Anatomical, histological and roentgenographic studies. *Journal of Bone and Joint Surgery,* **60A,** 575–85.

Putti V. (1933) Early treatment of congenital dislocation of the hip. *Journal of Bone and Joint Surgery,* **15,** 16.

Record R. G. & Edwards J. H. (1958) Environmental influences related to the aetiology of congenital dislocation of the hip. *British Journal of Preventitive and Social Medicine,* **12(1),** 8–22.

Roser W. (1864) Die Lehre von den Spontanluxationen. *Archives für Heilk,* **5,** 543.

Salter R. B. (1961) Innominate osteotomy in the treatment of congenital dislocation and subluxation of the hip. *Journal of Bone and Joint Surgery,* **43B,** 518.

Salter R. B., Kostuik J. & Dallas S. (1969) Avascular necrosis of the femoral head as a complication of treatment of congenital dislocation of the hip in young children. *Canadian Journal of Surgery,* **12,** 44–9.

Scott J. C. (1953) Frame reduction in congenital dislocation of the hip. *Journal of Bone and Joint Surgery,* **35B,** 372.

Severin E. (1941) Contribution to the knowledge of congenital dislocation of the hip joint. *Acta Chirurgica Scandinavica,* [Suppl] **84,** 63.

Smith W. S., Badgley C. E., Orwig J. B. & Harper J. M. (1968) Correlation of post-reduction roentgenograms and 31 year follow-up in congenital dislocation of the hip. *Journal of Bone and Joint Surgery,* **50A,** 1081–98.

Somerville E. W. & Scott J. C. (1957) The direct approach to congenital dislocation of the hip. *Journal of Bone and Joint Surgery,* **39B,** 623.

Somerville E. W. (1982) *Displacement of the Hip in Childhood.* Springer-Verlag, Berlin, Heidelberg, New York, Tokyo.

Steel H. H. (1977) Triple osteotomy of the innominate bone. *Clinical Orthopaedics,* **122,** 116–27.

Sutherland D. H. & Greenfield R. (1977) Double innominate osteotomy. *Journal of Bone and Joint Surgery,* **59A,** 1082.

Tachdjian M. O. (ed.) (1982) *Congenital Dislocation of the Hip.* Churchill Livingstone, New York, Edinburgh, London, Melbourne.

Tönnis D. (1976) Normal values of the hip joint for the evaluation of X-rays in children and adults. *Clinical Orthopaedics,* **119,** 39–47.

Trendelenburg F. (1895) Uber den Gang bei der angeborenen Hüftverrenkung. *Deutsche Medizinische Wochenschrift,* **21,** 21.

Trueta J. (1957) The normal vascularity of the human femoral head during growth. *Journal of Bone and Joint Surgery,* **39B,** 358–67.

Vickers R. H. & Catterall A. (1980) A trial of closed reduction: a method of management in congenital dislocation of the hip under the age of 2. *Journal of Bone and Joint Surgery,* **62B,** 526.

von Rosen S. (1962) Diagnosis and treatment of congenital dislocation of the hip joint in the newborn. *Journal of Bone and Joint Surgery,* **44B,** 284.

Wagner H. (1978) Experiences with spherical acetabular osteotomy for the correction of the dysplastic acetabulum. In *Acetabular Dysplasia; Skeletal Dysplasia in Childhood,* pp. 131–145. *Progress in Orthopaedic Surgery,* 2nd ed. U. H. Weil, Springer, New York.

Wainwright D. (1976) The shelf operation for hip dysplasia in adolescence. *Journal of Bone and Joint Surgery,* **58B,** 159.

Weinberg H. & Pogrund H. (1980) Effect of pelvic inclination on the pathogenesis of congenital hip dislocation. *Israeli Journal of Medical Science,* **16(4),** 229–33.

Weintroub S., Green I., Terdiman R. & Weissman S. L. (1979) Growth and development of congenitally dislocated hips reduced in early infancy. *Journal of Bone and Joint Surgery,* **61A,** 125–30.

Weintroub S., Boyd A., Chrispin R. A. & Lloyd-Roberts G. C. (1981) The use of stereophotogrammetry to measure acetabular and femoral anteversion. *Journal of Bone and Joint Surgery,* **63B,** 209.

Wiberg G. (1939) Studies on dysplastic acetabula and congenital subluxation of the hip joint with special reference to the complication of osteoarthritis. *Acta Chirurgica Scandinavica,* **58,** 83.

Wilkinson J. A. (1963) Prime factors in the aetiology of congenital dislocation of the hip. *Journal of Bone and Joint Surgery,* **45B,** 268.

Wilkinson J. A. (1985) *Congenital Displacement of the Hip Joint.* Springer-Verlag, Berlin, Heidelberg, New York, Tokyo.

Wilson J. C. (1974) Surgical treatment of the dysplastic acetabulum in adolescence. *Clinical Orthopaedics,* **98,** 137.

Wynne-Davies R. (1970a) Acetabular dysplasia and familial joint laxity: Two aetiological factors in congenital dislocation of the hip. A review of 589 patients and their families. *Journal of Bone and Joint Surgery,* **52B,** 704.

Wynne-Davies R. (1970b) A family study of neonatal and late-diagnosis congenital dislocation of the hip. *Medical Genetics,* **7,** 315.

5

The Irritable Hip

G. C. BENNET

The term irritable hip implies a symptom complex rather than a specific disease. Whilst it may result from one of several disorders considered elsewhere in this book, we will examine in detail one cause, namely transient synovitis. Whether this is in fact a specific disease is itself open to question. It has an importance greater than the pathological process might suggest for two reasons: first it is undoubtedly the commonest cause of hip pain in children (Caravias 1956) and secondly it may mimic the early stages of other, more serious, hip complaints. It was first recorded as long ago as 1892 by Lovett and Morse who described 'a short lived and ephemeral form of hip disease' due to 'simple acute synovitis'. For many years its importance lay in its differentiation from tuberculosis and undoubtedly many cases of transient synovitis were treated as such. Since that first description it has been known by a variety of names. These have included coxitis fugax, observation hip, transitory arthritis and acute transient epiphysitis which have all found favour at various times. The presently used term transient synovitis at least does not suggest any one aetiology and may indeed be a pathologically accurate description of the disease process. The multiplicity of names, however, merely emphasizes our ignorance of the condition and its underlying aetiology. This ignorance is understandable as it is a difficult disease to study. It has no specific signs or symptoms, there are no characteristic radiographic changes and laboratory investigations are of little help. Whilst the commonest cause of hip disability in childhood, its true incidence is unknown as many, perhaps the majority of mild cases, are not brought to medical attention as the symptoms are so minor and short lived.

Aetiology

The aetiology remains obscure. Trauma, allergy and infection, either bacterial or viral, have all been suspected, but the supporting evidence for any one of these is unconvincing.

There is no doubt that trauma can produce the clinical picture of transient synovitis. In such cases there is a history of a significant injury followed either immediately, or within a short space of time, by the onset of hip symptoms. If the hip is aspirated blood or clear fluid under pressure is obtained. More commonly, however, there is only a vague recollection of minor trauma usually some days previously. Whether such a history is of any significance is doubtful. Perhaps the main reason for trauma being implicated is that boys, who are presumed to be more vigorous, are more often affected than girls. Additionally, the age group affected certainly corresponds to the period when children are most liable to sustain minor trauma. Hardinge (1970) compared the seasonal variation of transient synovitis on the one hand with that of fractures of the tibia on the other, the presumption being that if trauma were implicated in the aetiology of transient synovitis, its seasonal prevalence would mirror that of a condition which truly reflected the trauma sustained in the community, namely fractures of the tibia. While some similarity was present, the relationship was not statistically significant.

Because of the fleeting nature of the disease, the occasional accompanying low grade pyrexia and raised white cell count and the fact that resolution is usually complete, a viral aetiology has been suspected. Additionally, joint symptoms are a well known accompaniment of some childhood viral illnesses, for example rubella and mumps. On this basis systematic searches for a causative viral agent have been undertaken (Blockey & Porter 1968, Hardinge 1970). No evidence to support the hypothesis was found so that, whilst it is impossible to prove a negative, a viral aetiology appears unlikely.

Bacterial infection was long held to be the likeliest cause. The lack of permanent damage to the joint as a result of such infection was explained by suggesting that they were either low grade or very localized (Butler 1933, Finder 1936, Miller 1931). There is little evidence to support such a contention. No growth has ever been obtained on hip aspiration or biopsy (as a matter of semantics, if it were the diagnosis would of course be septic arthritis). The white cell count is seldom raised and antimicrobial therapy does not seem to alter the course of the disease.

Several authors (Edwards 1952, Rothschild et al. 1956) have proposed an allergic cause for the disease on the basis of a hypersensitivity reaction to infection elsewhere. Whilst undoubtedly a proportion of affected children have a history of allergic disease, this is no more commonly found in children with transient synovitis than in the general population (Nachemson & Scheller 1969). The same goes for a recent history of infection. Whilst stress has been put upon the high proportion of children in whom an attack of transient synovitis is preceded by an upper respiratory tract infection (Chung 1981) there is little evidence to support this. In a study of limping children (Illingworth 1978) it was found that, in the group where the cause for the limp was in the hip, 54% had had an upper respiratory tract infection whereas, in those in whom the cause for the limp lay elsewhere, that is the control group, 53% had been similarly affected.

Nor does there appear to be a particular group of children at risk of developing the disease. Unlike Legg–Calvé–Perthes disease which affects a similar age group, no relationship with social class, birth weight, skeletal maturity, small stature or renal tract abnormalities has been described.

Thus the aetiology remains obscure. There is no evidence to suggest that a single aetiological agent is responsible and rather, it seems much more likely that a variety of insults can produce the same symptom complex.

Pathology

Because of the benign nature of the condition only a limited amount of pathological material has become available for study. Such material as there is, is likely to have been obtained from the more severe part of the spectrum of the disease where the diagnosis was in doubt and, in consequence, the hip was either aspirated or explored. Aspiration usually produces a few millilitres of straw coloured fluid, sometimes under tension, which has no special characteristics and from which no growth is obtained on culture. Synovial biopsies have similarly been of limited value. All have shown nonspecific inflammatory changes but, as the synovium can react to an insult in a very limited number of ways, this lack of specificity is hardly surprising.

Experimental studies have yielded little information. Pathological changes similar to those found in transient synovitis have been produced by injecting talc into the hip joints of rabbits (Gershuni & Axer 1974). The injections caused synovial inflammation and hypertrophy. The resulting hyperaemia produced an increase in the size of the femoral head and thickening of the articular cartilage, the latter being evident radiographically as an increased medial joint space. In some experimental animals, the cartilage changes subsequently reverted to normal. Kemp (1973) produced changes similar to those of transient synovitis by instilling dextran into the hip joints of experimental animals. Whilst of interest, these experiments help little in the basic understanding of the disease and in particular whether it is the result of a response to a single entity rather than a nonspecific response to a variety of childhood accidents and ailments.

Clinical features

The disorder is most commonly found in children between the ages of two and ten with a peak between five and seven years. Boys are more commonly affected than girls in a ratio of 2:1. Both hips are equally affected and bilateral disease is rare. The onset may be acute or chronic with around half presenting in each way. In the acute form the child will often awaken in the morning and refuse to weightbear on the affected leg. In such cases they seldom localize the site of the discomfort. In the older child, limp and pain of variable severity predominate. As in other childhood disorders it should not be forgotten that pain emanating from the hip may be referred to the ipsilateral thigh or knee. When the onset is acute, particularly in the younger child who refuses to weightbear, medical attention is usually sought at an early stage, whereas in the case of the older child with a limp, but little pain, the initial symptoms may be met with parental suspicion and consequently delay in seeking medical advice is common.

Examination usually reveals a well looking, albeit often apprehensive child, of whom around 25% will have a low grade pyrexia. The affected hip is normally held in some degree of flexion, abduction and external rotation. This is the position of maximum comfort in the presence of a joint effusion, as it corresponds to the position of maximum joint volume and thus that of least pressure (Eyring & Murray 1964). Palpation anterior to the hip often reveals some slight tenderness. The Trendelenberg sign may be positive, presumably on an antalgic basis. Muscle wasting is not a feature of this disease and its presence should be taken as an indication of there being some other cause for the child's symptoms. Movements of the hip are limited by a variable amount ranging from mild restriction of abduction and internal rotation to acute spasm of a severity to mimic that found in septic arthritis.

Differential diagnosis

The early stages of several hip disorders are characterized by acute synovitis and it may be clinically impossible to differentiate them from transient synovitis. Legg–Calvé–Perthes disease is perhaps the commonest cause of this problem, but early septic arthritis and tuberculosis can give rise to similar difficulties. Chronic synovitis can usually only be diagnosed with confidence retrospectively when the anticipated resolution of the disease does not occur.

Fractures, slipped capital femoral epiphysis, tumour or leukaemic deposits are all less common conditions to be excluded.

Investigations

A full blood count and an erythrocyte sedimentation rate (ESR) should always be performed. Haematological abnormalities such as leukaemia can then be excluded. A white cell count is useful in differentiating transient synovitis from septic arthritis, as in the former it is usually normal (Adams 1963) whereas in the latter a marked rise is almost invariable. The differentiation is further helped by the ESR which in septic arthritis is raised, often to very high levels, whereas the opposite is true in transient synovitis. Adams (1963) found only five of fifty cases of transient synovitis had an ESR of more than 20 and this reflects the general experience.

The other mainstay of investigation is the plain radiograph. Whilst is may show an increased medial joint space (Fig. 5.1) it is more usually helpful in exluding other conditions rather than making a positive diagnosis of transient synovitis. In Legg–Calvé–Perthes disease the initial radiograph is abnormal in 90% (Adams 1963). Slipped capital femoral epiphysis, fractures and tumours can be excluded with at least the same degree of confidence. Much has been made of the soft tissue changes supposedly found in synovitis (Fox & Griffin 1956). The capsular shadow is characteristically said to be displaced laterally, this being taken as a sign of the presence of an effusion in the hip joint. Additionally the soft tissue shadow between the glutei and that outlining the psoas are both said to be blurred in the presence of inflammation (Neuhauser & Wittenburg 1963). These signs, however, have been discredited by Brown (1975) who demonstrated that the appearance of capsular distension was dependent upon the position of the hip. Specifically, the capsule appeared distended when the hip was laterally rotated and abducted, exactly the position adopted by the child with transient synovitis. He further showed, this time in a cadaveric study, that the X-ray shadow usually thought to be produced by the capsule does in fact represent an intermuscular tissue plane starting anteriorly between sartorius and tensor fascia lata and extending back beyond the hip.

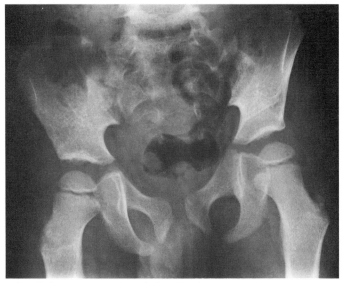

Fig. 5.1 Increased medial joint space in the right hip. This boy sustained a significant injury to the hip 48 hours before admission.

Other investigations have been used in a small number of cases. Gershuni *et al.* (1978) reported the results of arthrograms performed in three cases of transient synovitis. In each of the three an increase in head size was found and in two an increased medial joint space was an additional finding. Ultrasound has been shown to be an accurate way of diagnosing a hip joint effusion (Wingstrad 1984) to an extent that it can demonstrate a reduction in the volume of fluid present after aspiration.

Isotope scanning can be helpful in picking out the small number of children with Perthes disease who have a normal initial X-ray (Fig. 5.2). Positive or diagnostic findings specific to transient synovitis are once again lacking. Most indeed are normal. Carty *et al.* (1984) scanned 129 cases of transient synovitis and found 111 to be normal. Of the remainder, 16 had a diffusely increased uptake and 2 had a

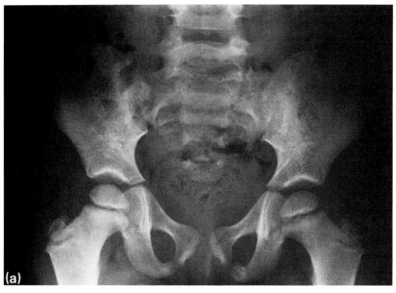

Fig. 5.2 (a) A six-year-old girl who presented with symptoms initially thought to be caused by transient synovitis of the left hip. Apart from regional osteoporosis, the radiographs showed no abnormality.

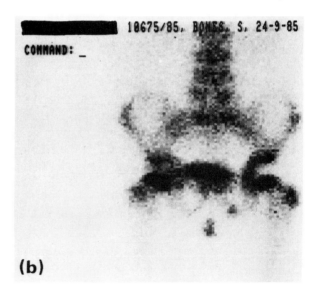

(b) The isotope scan, however, showed the typical changes of Perthes disease of the left hip.

similarly diffuse reduction, these presumably reflecting the decrease in blood flow secondary to the presence of an effusion. Similar findings have been reported by other authors (Herndon *et al.* 1985).

Management

In the vast majority of cases, the clinical picture, combined with the haematological investigations and plain radiograph suffice to make a confident diagnosis of transient synovitis. Bedrest is then usually advised. If the child is only mildly uncomfortable and social circumstances permit, then there is no reason why this should not take place at home. In such cases the advice given to parents should be realistic. There is no point in issuing a strict timetable for bedrest as it is almost impossible to keep an otherwise fit 6-year-old child in bed once he does not want to stay there. If the symptoms are rather more acute or there is doubt as to the diagnosis then admission to hospital should be advised. Whilst such children are usually put on bedrest with light skin traction, the rationale for this is obscure. There is no doubt that most children quickly settle on such a regime, but that is not to say that it is cause and effect. As we have already noted, children with a hip joint effusion adopt the position of maximum comfort namely, abduction, flexion and external rotation of the hip, this corresponding to the position of maximum volume of the joint. Extending the hip on traction will increase the intracapsular pressure and may, as a result, increase the discomfort. That said, however, there is no evidence that it has a deleterious effect. It would seem more logical, however, if traction is to be used, that it should be applied in some degree of flexion. An alternative to traction is the use of slings and springs which has the added advantage of allowing the child to move the hip within the limits of comfort.

Within two or three days the discomfort usually resolves and hip movement is regained, although some slight restriction, particularly of abduction and internal rotation, may remain. There seems little point in waiting for a complete return of motion and the child can usually be allowed out of bed at this point. If a marked limp remains or recurs, then a further period of bedrest is indicated. The vast majority have no such setback and can be allowed home after 24 hours unrestricted weightbearing.

The place of any more active therapy is questionable. Antibiotics have often been used, not so much for the primary condition, as for the treatment of associated, usually upper respiratory tract, infections. There is no evidence that they alter the course of the disease in any way. Certainly there is no justification for their empirical use should there be doubt as to the diagnosis. Antihistamines (Edwards 1952) and cortisone (Rothschild et al. 1956) have both been given on the basis that the disease has an allergic basis. Although claims as to their efficacy have been made, their use has not received any widespread support nor have any trials been undertaken. Their effects must remain anecdotal and highly questionable.

In the relatively small proportion of children who present with severe restriction of movement, there may be difficulty in excluding hip joint sepsis. In those cases aspiration of the joint, almost invariably under general anaesthesia, is indicated. Even when no infected material is found, removal of some of the joint effusion in these more severe cases often results in a remarkable resolution of symptoms such that, when the child recovers from the anaesthetic, spasm is minimal and an excellent range of movement can be obtained.

Subsequent course

The vast majority of children settle on such simple measures, but in a proportion the symptoms and signs grumble on. In them the diagnosis should be reviewed as they may be suffering from chronic, rather than acute, synovitis.

In those that do settle as anticipated, the parents should be warned of two possible late complications, namely recurrence and Perthes disease. In a review of the literature Illingworth (1983) found that 17.4% of cases recurred. Whilst the majority of cases in her series did so within the first year, in a sizeable minority the recurrence did not take place until the second and in some it was considerably later. The early course of the disease gave no clue as to which children were likely to develop a recurrence. In another study of recurrent transient synovitis (Jacobs 1971) 11 of 18 children were subsequently found to have Perthes disease.

The relationship of transient synovitis to Perthes disease is difficult to determine. The two disorders have much in common. The initial presentation is similar, they occur in the same age group and both are more common in boys. On that basis it is at least reasonable to suspect that they are in some way related. Certainly most published series of transient synovitis include a proportion of children who later prove to have, or develop Perthes disease, the actual percentage varying from 4–18% (Hardinge 1970, Jacobs 1971, Vandeputte *et al.* 1971). It would appear likely however that at least some cases were initially wrongly diagnosed and were not transient synovitis, but Perthes disease from the outset. Obviously, the more vigorously the diagnosis is sought in the first instance, for example by isotope scanning, the lower will be the proportion who later prove to have Perthes disease.

A relationship might also be expected on pathophysiological grounds. Perthes disease results in osteonecrosis of the femoral head as a result of an interruption to its blood supply. In transient synovitis fluid is present within the capsule of the hip joint and it may be hypothesized that this could cause such an interruption. It will be remembered that the epiphyseal plate forms a barrier to metaphyseal vessels reaching the capital epiphysis and that, until about the age of 10, the artery to the ligamentum teres plays no appreciable role in its blood supply. Thus, before that age the femoral head is reliant upon the ascending cervical branches of the lateral and medial circumflex femoral arteries. These run a subsynovial course within the capsule so that the flow in them is sensitive to intracapsular pressure. Numerous attempts have been made to reproduce Perthes disease experimentally by raising the intracapsular pressure. The results are rather contradictory for, although there is no doubt that a high enough pressure sustained for a long enough period will indeed have this effect, the relevance of these findings to the development of Perthes disease is questionable. Woodhouse (1964) found that a pressure of 50 mm of mercury sustained for 12 hours produced avascular necrosis in the femoral heads of dogs. Using a microsphere technique to measure blood flow, Lucht *et al.* (1983) demonstrated a 35% reduction in flow to the femoral head when the intracapsular pressure was maintained between venous and arterial. On the other hand Tachdjian & Grana (1968) found they could not produce avascular necrosis unless the intracapsular pressure was maintained above arterial. As it is known that in human subjects an intracapsular pressure as low as 20 mm H_2O can produce very marked pain (Gershuni *et al.* 1983) it seems unlikely that the often mild discomfort of transient synovitis is associated with very high pressure. The question of the relationship of transient synovitis to the later development of Perthes disease remains unresolved.

What of the ultimate fate of a hip affected by transient synovitis? Few longterm studies have been undertaken. On reviewing 50 cases followed up for between 1 and 15 years, Adams (1963) found 9 not to be radiographically normal, although none had any changes which suggested progression was likely. Nachemson & Scheller (1969) in perhaps the most complete follow-up examined 73 cases 20–22 years after their initial episode and compared them to an age matched control group. Only 1 of the 73 had had hip pain severe enough to warrant medical attention. Although 18 of the 67 examined had some limitation of motion of the hip, it was never by more than 20° (in 3 cases such limitation was found in the opposite 'normal' hip). The only significant radiological finding was an increased incidence of coxa magna as compared to the control group and they concluded that radiological sequelae were few and, if present, relatively mild.

References

Adams J. A. (1963) Transient synovitis of the hip joint in children. *Journal of Bone and Joint Surgery,* **45,** 471–6.

Blockey N. J. & Porter B. (1968) Transient synovitis of the hip. *British Medical Journal,* **4,** 557–8.

Brown I. (1975) A study of the 'capsular' hip shadow in disorders of the hip in children. *Journal of Bone and Joint Surgery,* **57B,** 175–9.

Butler R. W. (1933) Transitory arthritis of the hip joint in children. *British Medical Journal,* **1,** 951–4.

Caravias D. E. (1956) The significance of the so-called 'irritable hips' in children. *Archives of Disease in Childhood,* **31,** 415–8.

Carty H., Maxted M., Fielding J. A., Gulliford P. & Owen R. (1984) Isotope scanning in the irritable hip syndrome. *Skeletal Radiology,* **11,** 32–7.

Chung S. (1981) *Hip Disorders in Infants and Children,* pp. 269–73. Lea & Febiger, Philadelphia.

Edwards E. G. (1952) Transient synovitis of the hip joint in children. *Journal of the American Medical Association,* **148,** 30–4.

Eyring E. T. & Murray W. R. (1964) The Effect of joint position on the pressure of an intra-articular effusion. *Journal of Bone and Joint Surgery,* **46,** 235–41.

Finder J. G. (1936) Transitory synovitis of the hip joint in childhood. *Journal of the American Medical Association,* **107,** 3–5.

Fox K. W. & Griffin L. L. (1956) Transient synovitis of the hip joint in children. *Texas State Medical Journal,* **52,** 15–20.

Gershuni D. H. & Axer A. (1974) Synovitis of the hip joint — an experimental model in rabbits. *Journal of Bone and Joint Surgery,* **56B,** 59–77.

Gershuni D. H., Axer A. & Hendel D. (1978) Arthrographic findings in Legg–Calvé–Perthes disease and transient synovitis of the hip. *Journal of Bone and Joint Surgery,* **60A,** 457–64.

Gershuni D. H., Hargens A. R., Lee Y. F., Greenberg E. N., Zapf R. & Akeson W. H. (1983) The questionable significance of hip joint tamponade in producing osteonecrosis in Legg–Calvé–Perthes Disease. *Journal of Pediatric Orthopedics,* **3,** 280–6.

Hardinge K. (1970) The aetiology of transient synovitis of the hip in children. *Journal of Bone and Joint Surgery,* **52B,** 100–7.

Herndon W. A., Alexieva B. J., Schwindt M. L., Scott K. N. & Hafferwo S. (1985) Nuclear imaging for musculoskeletal infections in children. *Journal of Pediatric Orthopedics,* **5,** 343–7.

Illingworth C. M. (1978) 128 limping children with no fracture, sprain or obvious cause. *Clinical Paediatrics,* **17,** 139–42.

Illingworth C. M. (1983) Recurrences of transient synovitis of the hip. *Archives of Disease in Childhood,* **58,** 620–3.

Jacobs B. W. (1971) Synovitis of the hip in children and its significance. *Pediatrics,* **47,** 558–66.

Kemp H. B. S. (1973) Perthes' disease: an experimental and clinical study. *Annals of the Royal College of Surgeons of England,* **52,** 18.

Lovett R. W. & Morse J. L. (1892) A transient ephemeral form of hip disease with a report of cases. *Boston Medical Journal,* **127,** 161–3.

Lucht C. Bunger B., Krebs B. & Bulow J. (1983) Blood flow changes in the juvenile hip in relation to changes of the intra-articular pressure. *Acta Orthopaedica Scandinavica,* **54,** 182–7.

Miller O. L. (1931) Acute transient epiphysitis of the hip joint. *Journal of the American Medical Association,* **96,** 575–9.

Nachemson A. & Scheller S. (1969) A clinical and radiological follow-up study of transient synovitis of the hip. *Acta Orthopaedica Scandinavica,* **40,** 479–500.

Neuhauser E. & Wittenburg M. (1963) Synovitis of the Hip in Infancy and Childhood. *Radiologic Clinics of North America,* **1,** 13–6.

Rothschild H. B., Russ J. D. & Wasserman C. F. (1956) Corticotrophins in the treatment of transient synovitis of the hip in children. *Journal of Pediatrics,* **49,** 33–7.

Tachjdian M. O. & Grana L. (1968) Response of the hip joint to increased intra-articular pressure. *Clinical Orthopaedics,* **61,** 199–212.

Vandeputte L. Mulier C. & Mulier F. (1971) Transient synovitis of the hip joint in children. *Acta Orthopaedica Belgica,* **37,** 186–93.

Wingstrad H. (1984) Ultrasonography in hip joint effusion: report of a child with transient synovitis. *Acta Orthopaedica Scandinavica,* **55,** 469–71.

Woodhouse C. F. (1964) Dynamic influences in vascular occlusion affecting the development of avascular necrosis of the femoral head. *Clinical Orthopaedics,* **32,** 119–29.

6

The Infected Hip

M. G. H. SMITH

As infection of the child's hip may involve bony sites and as purely bony infection may mimic hip joint infection, pelvic and femoral neck osteitis will be considered along with the hip joint, both in acute and chronic infections.

Acute infection

With the rare exception of direct implantation in the course of femoral venepuncture in the very young carried out with inadequate aseptic technique (Chacha 1971), infection of the hip joint or its immediate surroundings is blood borne.

Whether the infection involves the synovium directly or a bony site close to the joint with secondary spread, the early course for the joint is the same. The results will depend upon the severity of the infection, the delay in diagnosis and consequent delay in starting effective antibiotic treatment, with or without surgery, at all ages. The age of the child has a profound influence on the outcome as the diagnosis is likely to be delayed in the neonate and young infant and the young child's hip is more vulnerable to damage. Older children, able to complain of local pain and to demonstrate a limp or inability to walk, are usually brought to medical attention sooner so that delay in diagnosis is less likely. At any age geographic remoteness from hospital may be an important cause of delay in treatment.

At all ages infection is most likely to be due to staphylococcus aureus (88%, Blockey & McAllister 1972) with streptococcal and other infections accounting for only a small proportion. Although haemophilus infection is important in the age group six months to three years in other sites, it is seldom the causative organism in the hip.

Children with hip infection fall into two distinct groups:

1 The neonate and young infant who present with gross pathology, abscess formation and pathological dislocation late in the course of infection, perhaps one or two weeks after its onset.
2 Older children presenting early after 24–48 hours of infection without gross changes.

In both groups the diagnosis is primarily clinical based upon the awareness of the possibility of such infection. Laboratory and radiographic investigations are of secondary importance. The problems of these two groups will be taken separately.

Septic arthritis of the hip in the neonate and young infant

There may have been general illness of some, even many, days and the baby may have begun treatment in another speciality for a known or suspected infection such as septicaemia or for a focus of infection such as the umbilical stump. The baby is ill, often vomiting, but there may be little pyrexia. In the late presentation the ESR is likely to be high, with polymorphonuclear leucocytosis but neither of these features is invariably present.

It is the reduction of active movement of the part (pseudoparalysis) that is often the first indication of hip infection. The hip lies in flexion and attempts to move it passively in any direction, but particularly rotation, are resisted. Tenderness elicited by the distress of palpation, local swelling even to the point of gross distension of the buttock and evidence of frank dislocation of the hip are found in the later stages of the pathological course. A search for other sites of sepsis should be made so that local treatment appropriate to them can also be planned.

The radiographic features depend upon how advanced the infection may be. Initially there will be evidence of joint distension with increase in the soft tissue shadow of the joint capsule, an increase in the distance between the medial femoral metaphyseal corner and the medial wall of the acetabulum proceeding to frank lateral displacement of the femur and to actual dislocation, which usually occurs posteriorly, with the shadow of soft tissue swelling increasing with the clinical distension. After 7–10 days, evidence of bone erosion and periosteal bone formation may be present in the femoral metaphysis or part of the pelvis if the primary focus of infection is there (Figs. 6.1 & 6.2).

The result of the ESR and the white cell count need not be awaited. Treatment should start without delay apart from resuscitation of the very ill child with i.v. fluid, blood transfusion, etc. A blood culture must be carried out.

In the unusual event of an early diagnosis of septic arthritis in this age group, with no evidence of subluxation of the hip, simple aspiration of the joint will suffice to confirm the presence of purulent fluid and to obtain a specimen for bacteriological study. It is wise to immobilize the hip in an abduction plaster.

In the more usual situation of gross joint distension, perhaps associated with dislocation and buttock abscess formation, operation is needed to evacuate the pus. This is usually done via a posterior approach through the buttock. The abscess is easily found, emptied and followed down to the distended, ruptured joint capsule and dislocated femoral head. In severe cases the head may be partially absorbed or detached from the neck. The head, or what may be left of it, should be reduced, the wound closed with drainage and the hip immobilized in whatever position of abduction gives the most stable reduction.

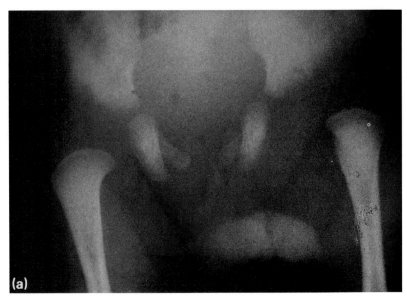

Fig. 6.1 (a) A male neonate unwell for two weeks has septic arthritis of the left hip. The hip is dislocated. Some erosion of the roof of the acetabulum indicates the site of the infection.

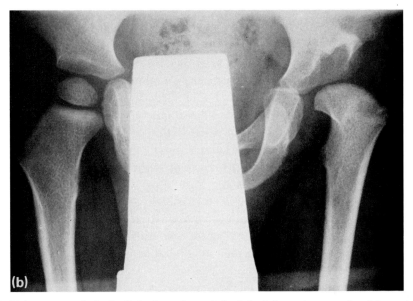

Fig 6.1. (b) At two years the leg is a little short, the capital epiphysis has not appeared and the acetabulum is defective. Function and movement are almost normal.

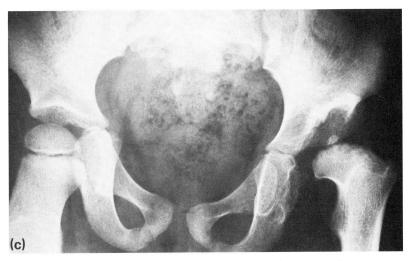

Fig. 6.1 (c) At five years the capital epiphysis has appeared.

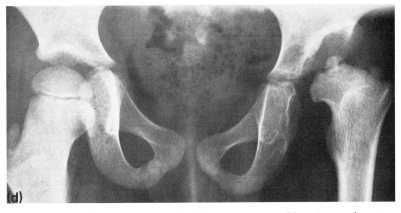

Fig. 6.1 (d) At seven years the leg remains short but movements and function are almost normal.

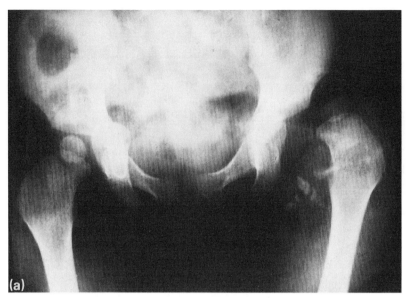

Fig. 6.2 (a) A female infant of nine months, presenting late after one or two weeks of upper left femoral osteitis. Periosteal new bone is apparent and the hip is dislocated.

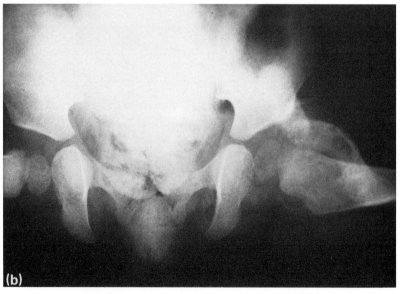

Fig. 6.2 (b) Aged one year, after drainage, reduction of hip and maintaining abduction in a 'frog' position plaster, the hip joint is satisfactory but a bar of ectopic bone joins the pelvis to the femur on its posterolateral aspect. This bar was then excised.

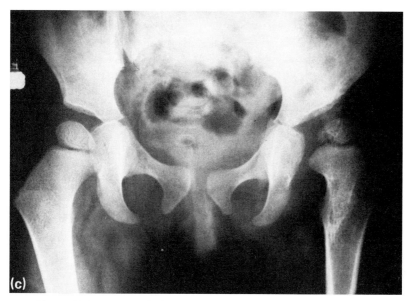

Fig. 6.2 (c) At two years the hip is dysplastic but clinically almost normal.

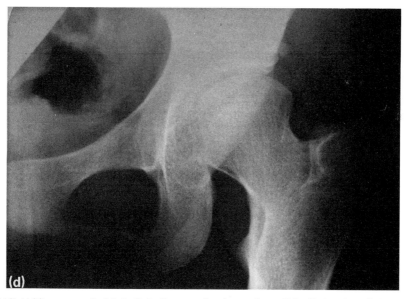

Fig. 6.2 (d) At fifteen years the hip is clinically normal and apart from slight diminution of joint space and the presence of a small bony fragment above the acetabulum the X-ray is now normal.

Antibiotics are given in generous dosage initially by the i.v. route, but oral administration may suffice. It may be anticipated that the bacteriologist will report in two or three days' time that staphyloccus aureus is the infecting organism so the appropriate antibiotic chosen on the 'best guess' would be cloxacillin given in a dosage of not less than 100 mg/kg/day in four doses. Should an unusual infection (for example *E. coli*) be suspected, a broader spectrum antibiotic should be chosen. (It is wise to keep the 'best guess' choice of antibiotics under review in one's clinical practice, with the advice of the bacteriologist as both the infecting organisms and their sensitivities may change with the passage of time.)

The duration of antibiotic treatment will generally be about 21 days but may be extended as long as needed if evidence of continuing infection exists. The use of plaster to maintain the abduction position of reduction should be continued for one or two months or until such time as redislocation seems unlikely.

As plasters are changed, evidence of stiffness in abduction should be looked for and less severely abducted positions applied. Local pelvic or femoral chronic osteitis may require sequestrectomy or curettage should such a focus later become evident.

Complications

The complications of septic arthritis of the hip in the baby are more common and more severe than in the older child.

Stability of the hip may be lost if the hip is not adequately reduced and held reduced. Late efforts to reduce the chronically dislocated hip have not proved to

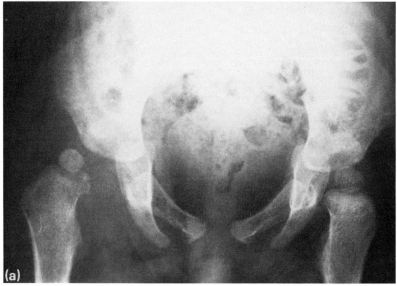

Fig. 6.3 (a) A female infant aged one year, treated elsewhere for a urinary infection has a subluxated right hip.

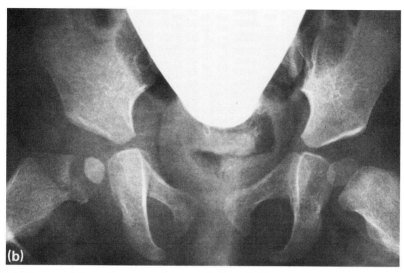

Fig. 6.3 (b) One month later after open arthrotomy the hip is held reduced in abduction plasters. The femoral capital epiphysis is avascular and radiologically denser than the surrounding bones and there is a metaphyseal erosion. No growth was obtained from the joint at exploration presumably due to the earlier antibiotics.

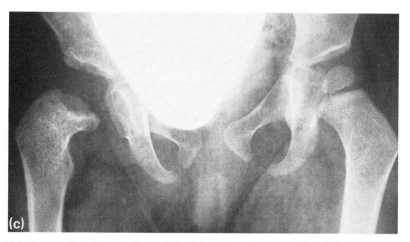

Fig. 6.3 (c) At one and a half years, the capital epiphysis has disappeared but the hip remains stable and has an almost full range of movement.

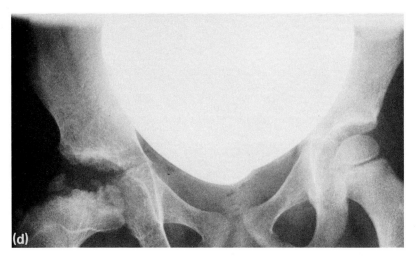

Fig. 6.3 (d) At four and a half years, the capital epiphysis is appearing with osteochondritic changes. There is slight shortening of the leg.

be rewarding. Rarely complications may occur in the efforts to maintain reduction in abduction for two months or longer as fibrosis or (exceptionally) ectopic bone formation develops in the soft tissues lateral to the hip producing fixation in the abducted position. This may necessitate surgery to restore the hip movements (Fig. 6.2).

Impairment of blood supply to the femoral capital epiphysis may occur due to the relatively critical vascular supply being exposed to the pressure of joint fluid and the inflammatory process within the joint. It is common for the capital epiphysis not to appear in X-rays as expected at about six months of age or, if already visible, to disappear over the months after infection. This leaves the surgeon not knowing if the head has been lost permanently or whether it will reappear over the course of the next year or two. If the head does reappear, a hip joint is obtained in which function is relatively normal although some loss of movement and femoral length may be present (Figs. 6.1 & 6.3). If, however, the head has been lost permanently the hip will not stabilize as the femur will migrate upwards resulting in a short poorly functioning limb (Fig. 6.4). This situation is best dealt with by trying to achieve stability, or possibly hip fusion, by putting the surviving trochanteric portion of the femur into the acetabulum.

The observation by Wientroub *et al.* (1981) that evidence of damage to or fusion of the triradiate cartilage indicated an absent or fused, useless femoral head in the acetabulum, is a useful pointer in that, if this sign is present, there is no point in delaying surgery to achieve stability.

On the re-appearance of the head, often with osteochondritic appearances (Fig. 6.3) the hip may return to a semblance of normality but if pseudoarthrosis of the neck is apparent and persists, this may require intertrochanteric osteotomy with

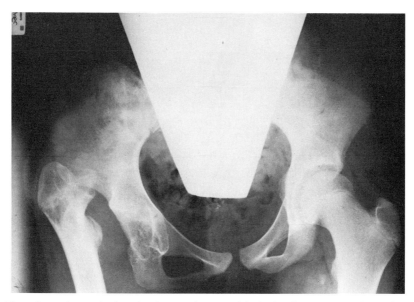

Fig. 6.4 The pelvic radiograph of a girl at the age of 15 years who had suffered septic arthritis of the right hip in infancy. There is now marked shortening and some stiffness.

medial displacement of the femoral shaft beneath the head to achieve union and stability (Fig. 6.5).

Septic arthritis of the hip in the older child

The course of the disease before diagnosis is much shorter than in the baby as the ability to localize and complain of pain and demonstrate a limp or inability to bear weight, leads to an early diagnosis, commonly within 24–48 hours. The diagnosis is essentially clinical. The child will be ill and usually pyrexial. Although pain may be referred to thigh or knee, examination will quickly locate pathology to the hip. *All* movement will be limited, especially rotation, with pain and muscle spasm. The hip may lie in some flexion, abduction and external rotation and local tenderness over the joint is usually found.

A search for a possible site of osteitis in the upper femur or in the pelvis should be carried out by local palpation, including rectal examination if the ischium is suspect.

X-rays at this stage will show no abnormality other than possible capsular distension and an increase in the medial clear space of the joint indicating the presence of a joint effusion. One to two weeks later a focus of osteitis in the femoral neck or pelvis may be seen if that has been the primary focus of infection.

The ESR is likely to be raised but with early diagnosis may not be very high. There is usually a polymorphonuclear leucocytosis. Neither of these features is essential to the diagnosis. Having made the presumptive diagnosis of septic

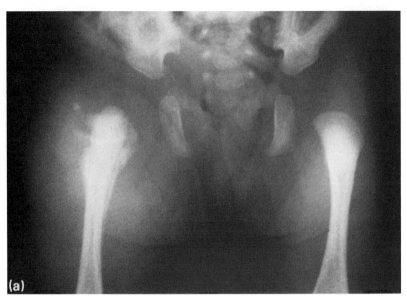

Fig. 6.5 (a) A female infant of six weeks treated elsewhere in the first two weeks of life for upper femoral osteitis. The changes about the upper femur are obvious but the hip is clinically and radiologically not involved or dislocated.

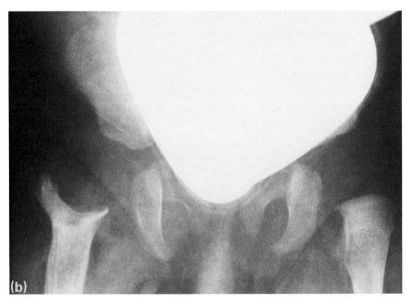

Fig. 6.5 (b) At four months there is severe distortion of the upper femur and neck region but the hip remains clinically normal.

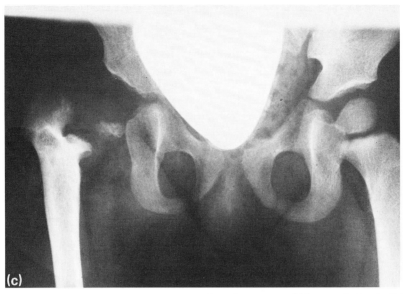

Fig. 6.5 (c) At two and a half years the capital epiphysis has appeared. The acetabulum is slightly dysplastic. The femoral neck may develop a pseudoarthrosis but is clinically intact. The greater trochanter is overgrowing and may need its growth stopped by epiphyseodesis.

arthritis, confirmation of this by joint fluid aspiration should be obtained. The nature of the fluid will help in the differential diagnosis and it should be submitted in blood culture bottles for bacteriological study.

The differential diagnosis in this situation includes the other following conditions:

1   noninfective synovitis of the hip which will later be proved to be transient but which is sufficiently marked to suggest possible septic arthritis;
2   acute traumatic haemarthrosis;
3   Henoch Schonlein purpura (HSP);
4   acute onset juvenile rheumatoid arthritis (JRA);
5   osteitis of pelvis not directly involving the hip.

Aspiration under general anaesthetic is best done from an anterosuperolateral approach from a site a little medial to the midpoint between the anterior superior iliac spine and the greater trochanter, aiming for the anterosuperior aspect of the proximal femoral neck (Fig. 6.6). On reaching the bone the needle tip should be within the joint capsule. With early diagnosis, even in the older child it is unusual to obtain more than 4–5 ml of fluid.

An acute traumatic haemarthrosis will be suspected from the child's history of trauma and if bloodstained fluid is aspirated. This in itself will be therapeutic. Under these circumstances bed rest with light traction should be sufficient treatment. If frankly bloodstained fluid is obtained without a history of trauma the

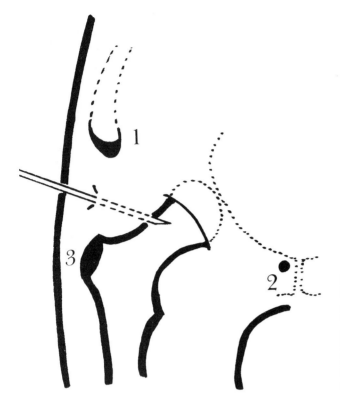

Fig. 6.6 Aspiration of the hip. The bony landmarks are: (1) The anterior superior iliac spine. (2) The pubic tubercule. (3) The greater trochanter. A disposable 19 gauge needle is suitable in all but the biggest children in whom longer needle is needed to reach the joint.

possibility of HSP should be considered and confirmation sought by searching for rashes, haematuria and the involvement of other joints. Help from a physician should be sought regarding management of this condition.

If not bloodstained but other than clear synovial fluid is obtained, the diagnosis of septic arthritis should be considered likely and treatment started. Treatment is bed rest with light traction (1 or 2 kilograms) in slight abduction. Antibiotics are given on the 'best guess' principle, the choice and dosage being the same as for the baby and infant.

Clinical resolution is usually obvious over the next few days. In the unusual event of failure to improve the possibility of an inappropriate choice of antibiotics should be considered and help from the fluid culture should be available in 2–3 days. The possibility of an unusual infection or of an alternative diagnosis (acute onset of JRA) must be contemplated and with this open arthrotomy and biopsy of the synovium considered.

In our experience it has not been necessary to perform an early arthrotomy in the early stages of the disease and we would not advocate this as a first line of treatment in all suspected cases of infection. This would lead to significant surgery and its attendant scar being inflicted upon cases of synovitis of the hip where simple aspiration can be carried out readily, harmlessly and just as informatively (Wilson & Di Paola 1986).

If later (one week or more), X-rays show evidence of osteitis of the femoral neck or pelvis, antibiotic treatment should continue for 21 days or more. If no evidence of bony infection is found and the clinical condition returns to normal, antibiotics may be stopped at 14 days, with cessation of traction and progressive mobilization being started.

In the uncomplicated case no radiological blemish may be found on follow-up over several years except for a small proportion who develop some degree of coxa magna. This is of no clinical significance. In the unusual event of a delay in diagnosis of 5 or 6 days or more, and with clinical evidence of distension of the joint, open arthrotomy and closed suction drainage if needed, is advised. Only in such late cases have serious complications occurred (Wilson & Di Paola 1986).

The complications in this latter situation are again those associated with interference with the blood supply to the femoral head. Within 3 months, X-rays may show Perthes-like changes with segmental collapse. The result is nearly always a severe distortion of the femoral head despite attempts to limit these with treatment along the lines of Perthes disease by stopping weightbearing or by the use of containment positions of abduction in plaster. Almost invariably permanent loss of movement and secondary osteoarthritis relatively early in adult life is the likely outcome. Rarely in the older child will the femoral head be absorbed and in this situation an effort to achieve stability by hip fusion should be made.

Chronic infection of the hip, pyogenic and tuberculous

In addition to chronic infection of the hip, chronic pyogenic osteitis of the pelvis must be considered. Blood borne infection of the innominate bone is a rare but troublesome condition. This rarity causes the possibility to be overlooked, with failure to detect the site of infection by local examination, especially in the more deeply placed parts of the pelvis. The child may already have had an abdominal exploration for suspected appendicitis or may have been treated for a time with antibiotics for supposed peritonitis. Radiographs do not show sites of bony erosion or periosteal new bone formation clearly due to the complex three dimensional structure of the pelvis with its overlying soft tissue and bony shadows of varying density.

The diagnosis is likely to remain in doubt until an abscess appears. When this is drained the infection is followed to a bony site. In the mainly cancellous bone of the pelvis multilocular abscesses occur. The eradication of such an infection is difficult as the extent of bone involvement is difficult to assess even if X-ray sinograms are performed or generous resection of bone is carried out. Longterm (months or years) antibiotic treatment, with perhaps a number of attempts at local clearance, may be needed before infection is eradicated.

Chronic infection of the hip joint

This is nearly always tuberculous in nature. Although now rare, the occurrence of tuberculosis must be kept in mind as early diagnosis and the appropriate treatment will lead to the joint being restored to normal. Delay entails the risk of permanent residual damage even after the infection is eradicated.

The tuberculous hip infection is secondary to a primary source in lung or glands in neck or abdomen. Any age other than the young infant may be affected. The incidence in the UK is much higher in immigrants of Asian origin.

As in other skeletal sites (other large joints, small bones of hands and feet and in the spine) the infection is characterized by slow progress, low grade symptoms and an ability to produce large 'cold' abscesses. At the hip the joint synovium or the pelvis close to the acetabulum becomes infected though blood spread.

Low grade pain, possibly referred to thigh or knee, associated stiffness and limp are the usual symptoms. If sufficiently advanced there may be wasting of buttock and thigh and a position of flexion, abduction and external rotation may initially be adopted. Nowadays it would be most unusual for the condition to be so advanced at presentation for the child to adopt the classical posture of flexion, adduction and internal rotation or to have 'starting pains', night sweats or discharging sinuses.

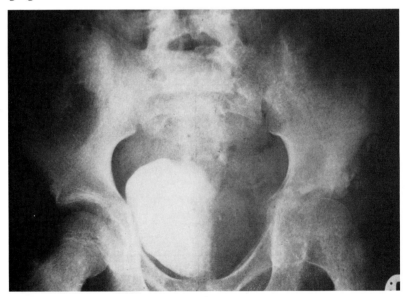

Fig. 6.7 A boy of 8 years had tuberculosis of the left hip for several months. There is general atrophic change about the hip, with evidence of erosion and periosteal new bone above and medial to the acetabulum. This IVP cystogram demonstrates the large intrapelvic 'cold' abscess that has developed without symptoms.

A mild pyrexia, an elevated ESR and a relative lymphocytosis in the blood picture would be expected but are not invariably present. With early presentation with a few rather nonspecific physical signs, the differential diagnosis includes:

1   Perthes disease;
2   slipped upper femoral epiphysis;
3   acute chondrolysis;
4   juvenile chronic (rheumatoid) arthritis;
5   chronic pyogenic pelvic osteitis.

The confirmation of diagnosis of tuberculosis rests upon four points:

1   the presence of a positive Mantoux test;
2   an X-ray appearance *consistent* with the diagnosis (this may be variable);
3   typical histology in infected material;*
4   culture of the tuberculous organism from infected material*

*These aspects require open biopsy.

X-rays including lateral views should be sufficient to confirm or deny the presence of Perthes disease or of slipped upper femoral epiphysis. In tuberculosis however, appearances are seldom diagnostic. Generalized bone atrophy in the region, narrowing of the joint space due to thinning of the articular cartilage and evidence of synovial thickening or joint effusion may all be features of acute chondrolysis or chronic rheumatoid arthritis. The radiological detection of a local area of bone destruction or a local abscess is very suggestive of tuberculosis as is a focus in the upper femoral metaphysis which crosses the epiphyseal plate to enter the capital epiphysis.

The only way that the diagnosis of tuberculosis can be confirmed or refuted is by biopsy, so obtaining material for histology and for bacterial culture. A certain diagnosis must be made so that the tuberculous child will not be left without treatment for an unnecessarily long time and conversely that a nontuberculous condition will not be subjected to inappropriate (and potentially toxic) drug treatment merely on the presumption of tuberculosis being present.

The diagnostic process may be combined very conveniently with therapy in that the opportunity can be taken to evacuate an abscess, curette out an osseous site or remove bulky inflamed synovium. Access can be from any approach, anterior, lateral, posterior or abdominal via the retroperitoneal space. Prior to biopsy investigation may include IVP (to screen for coexisting renal tuberculosis) and the cystogram from this may delineate an unsuspected pelvic abscess waiting to be drained (Fig. 6.7). It is customary to include sputum (or gastric washings) and urine specimens for bacteriological assessment of possible pulmonary or kidney infection.

From the time of biopsy antituberculous therapy should start (to be discontinued if the diagnosis is later discarded) and immobilization of the hip in a neutral position either by traction or in a hip spica for one to three months is undertaken.

The classic triad of streptomycin, isoniazid and para-aminosalicylic acid (PAS) has been shown to be effective over many years in the following dosage schedule (Hutchison 1980).

Streptomycin (IM) 40 mg/kg/day daily (stopping after 3 months)
Isoniazid 10–20 mg/kg/day in divided dosage
PAS 300 mg/kg/day in divided dosage

Bacteriological study of the biopsy material may show that the above regime is inappropriate and the following alternative regime may be used (Forfar & Arneil 1984):

Isoniazid 20 mg/kg/day in divided dosage
Rifampicin 25 mg/kg/day in divided dosage
Streptomycin 40 mg/kg/day daily (stopping after 3 months)

If the patient is not vomiting, streptomycin may be replaced by Ethambutol 25 mg/kg in a single daily oral dose.

These oral drugs should be continued for six months to one year.

With early diagnosis associated with little or no joint destruction, the aim is to produce a normal or nearly normal joint. As evidence of healing is seen in X-rays and as the ESR falls in the months following the start of treatment, mobilization and the progressive return to normal activity can be started.

If gross destruction of hip joint has occurred, ankylosis in a functional position may have to be accepted or a formal arthrodesis carried out.

References

Blockey N. J. & McAllister T. A. (1972) Antibiotics in acute osteomyelitis in children. *Journal of Bone and Joint Surgery*, **54B**, 299–309.

Chacha P. B. (1971) Suppurative arthritis of the hip joint in infancy — a persistent diagnostic problem and possible complication of femoral venepuncture. *Journal of Bone and Joint Surgery*, **53A**, 538–44.

Forfar J. O. & Arneil G. C. (1984) *Textbook of Paediatrics*, Third Edition, p. 403. Churchill Livingstone, Edinburgh.

Hutchison J. H. (1980) *Practical Paediatric Problems*, Fifth Edition, p. 76. Lloyd Luke (Medical Books) Ltd., London.

Wientroub S., Lloyd-Roberts G. C. & Fraser M. (1981) The prognostic significance of the triradiate cartilage in suppurative arthritis of the hip in infancy and early childhood. *Journal of Bone and Joint Surgery*, **63B**, 190–3.

Wilson N. I. L. & Di Paola M. (1986) Acute septic arthritis in infancy and childhood. *Journal of Bone and Joint Surgery*, **68B**, 584–7.

7

Perthes Disease

A. CATTERALL

Introduction

Although the literature on Perthes disease continues to increase the cause of this disease remains unknown. Preventive treatment is, therefore, impossible and management must be based on the endeavours of clinical examination and interpretation of radiological images. One of the main problems is the variable nature of the disease in which some 60% of patients do well without treatment. This suggests that a 'standard treatment' cannot be applied to every case.

Aetiology

The cause of this condition is unknown. In recent years, research by a number of different workers has suggested that there may be 'a susceptible child' to whom a subsequent incident occurs to the hip joint resulting in the radiological changes of Perthes disease. This concept is suggested for a number of reasons:

1   There is no evidence for an inherited abnormality in these children (Wynne-Davies & Gormley 1978).
2   80% of patients are between the age of 4 and 9 years with a sex ratio of 4:1 in favour of boys. This is increased to 7:1 in bilateral cases.
3   The incidence of this condition varies, being more common in the northwest region of England and in Scotland and in urban rather than rural communities. Within the city of Liverpool, Hall *et al.* (1983) have shown a variation in incidence from 0–29 cases per 10,000 and that this variability correlates with social class. On the basis of this evidence a nutritional cause for this condition is postulated.
4   There is strong evidence for environment factors with an increased chance of a child coming from families of low social class, and having low birth weight. Breech presentation is observed in 25% of cases during the last trimester of pregnancy (Hall *et al.* 1983, Wynne-Davis & Gormley 1978).
5 Inguinal hernia, genitourinary anomalies (Catterall 1971), and growth disturbances are common in these children. The growth disturbance is unusual in that it is disproportionate, the shortening involving the distal limbs hands and feet

(Burwell *et al.* 1978). Bone age is also delayed (Ralston 1955, Harrison *et al.* 1976) and up to three years of skeletal delay may be observed not only in the patients but also other siblings of a family (Harrison *et al.* 1976). A possible explanation for these observations may be found by observing differences in endochondral ossification in the uninvolved hip of unilateral cases when compared with normal controls (Catterall 1982).

Pathology

There are in the literature very few reports of the morphology of this condition in the early phases. From these reports the evidence suggests that there is thickening of the articular cartilage with infarction of the bony epiphysis which may in some cases involve only part of the epiphysis of the bone, while in others the whole of the epiphysis is involved (Catterall 1982, Fig. 7.1). In the majority of cases there is reason to believe that more than one episode of infarction has occurred (McKibbin & Ralis 1974, Inoue *et al.* 1976). In the dome of the epiphysis a trabecular fracture occurs producing an early loss of epiphyseal height. On fine detail radiography the epiphysis appears dense (Fig. 7.2b) partly due to trabecular fracture, and appositional new bone formation, but mainly because of calcification of the necrotic marrow. Once infarction has occurred a process of repair becomes established to revascularize the intact avascular trabeculae by the process of 'creeping substitution' and to remove the loose necrotic bone in the apex of the femoral head replacing it by fibrocartilage. This repair process produces the appearances of fragmentation (Fig. 7.2c). In the thickened articular cartilage the repair is by endochondral ossification occurring as a natural growth process from the surface of viable trabeculae and as islands of new bone formation in the thickened anterior and lateral articular cartilage which gradually enlarge and then fuse with the bony

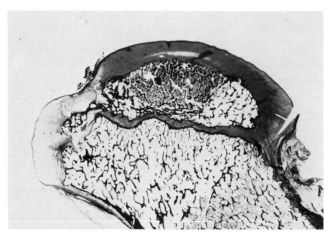

Fig. 7.1 Transverse section of central section of a Group II case. The articular cartilage is thickened. In the epiphysis the central area of infarction is noted with viable normal trabecular bone on its outer aspect. In the infarcted area the trabeculae are thickened and with evidence of trabecular fracture in the dome of the epiphysis producing loss of epipyseal height.

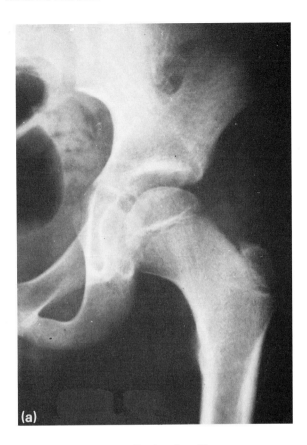

Fig. 7.2 The stages of the disease. (a) The phase of onset and anteroposterior radiograph showing increased density and widening of the inferomedial joint space. (*See* overleaf.)

(a)

epiphysis. Radiologically in the early stages these small islands of bone appear as areas of 'Calcification lateral to the epiphysis' and form one of the epiphyseal signs of the 'head at risk'. In the metaphysis, areas of unossified cartilage are seen streaming down from the growth plate producing the localized metaphyseal defect. Where these are large the normal architecture of the growth plate is lost and this means the growth of this part of the femoral neck is going to be abnormal. Because these lesions are usually anterolateral this will result in a growth disturbance in the femoral neck producing a tilt deformity of the femoral head on the neck.

The process of femoral head deformity

The preceding discussion has suggested that in the early phases of this disease there is a change in head shape due to overgrowth in articular cartilage with an overall loss of epiphyseal height due to trabecular fracture. This results in change of femoral head shape from round to oval. It is important to realize that this change occurs on both sides of the joint and that there is an early change in acetabular shape (Fig. 7.5) which is due to pressure of the femoral head on the edge of the lateral acetabular cartilage. Longterm remodelling, therefore, is 'off to a bad start'.

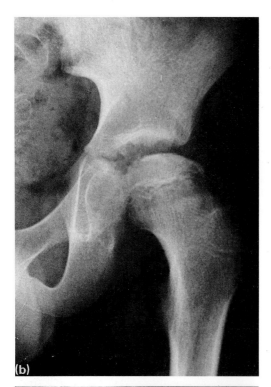

(b)

Fig 7.2 The stages of the disease.
(b)The phase of sclerosis. The
change in density compared with
(a) can be observed together with
alteration in the shape of the
epiphysis with loss of eipiphyseal
height. The increased density is
well seen, together with
reabsorption of the lateral aspect
of the epiphysis (Gage's sign). A
metaphyseal lesion is noted.

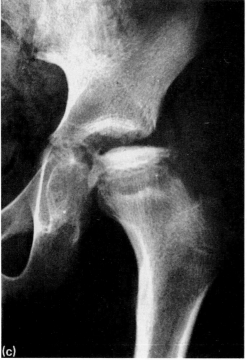

(c)

(c) The phase of fragmentation.
The lateral two-thirds of the
epiphysis is collapsed and is
being reabsorbed leaving an
intact and viable medial fragment
(Group III). There is lateral
uncovering of the femoral head
and the area to be reabsorbed has
a lucent zone medially to it. New
bone is noted lateral to the
collapsed segment.

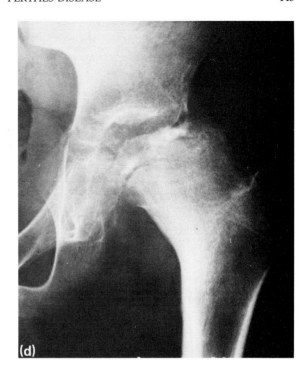

(d) The phase of healing. Healing is established with considerable deformity of the femoral head. There is an increase in size of the medial segment and in the size and quality of the bone forming in the thickened articular cartilage lateral to the original epiphysis.

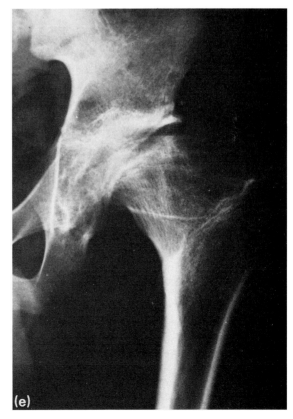

(e) The definitive phase. There is a coxa magna with deformity of the femoral head. The overall result is poor because of shortening of the femoral neck, uncovering of the femoral head and the relative high position of the greater trochanter. There is a transcervical line identifying the anterior extent of femoral head deformity.

In the longterm the femoral head remains either oval or progressively flattens to 'a roller bearing shape' in which there is an overgrowth of the flattened femoral head outside the acetabulum and the axis of movement is in the flexion/extension range only (Fig. 7.3). Because of the varus deformity of the femoral neck the leg lies adducted and is therefore short in extension with the axis of movement being from extension and adduction to flexion and abduction. The earliest changes of this process may be recognized clinically by a progressive loss of abduction and rotation and an alteration in the axis of flexion. Radiologically and arthrographically this alteration may be observed by loss of abduction and a change in its manner from one of pure rotation to rotation with hinging on the lateral aspect of the acetabulum. Once the moment of this hinging is outside the confines of the bony acetabulum the subluxation becomes fixed and the roller bearing joint is the inevitable result. This process is called 'hinge abduction' (Fig. 7.9).

It follows from this summary that if a round or oval femoral head is to be maintained a free range of movement must be maintained throughout the disease process. This will allow moulding of the biologically plastic articular cartilage. Once the bone islands coalesce within the lateral aspect the plasticity of this tissue is lost and subsequent change in the lateral aspect of the femoral head shape can only be achieved as the result of growth and remodelling.

Prognostic factors

In a disease in which 60% of cases do well without treatment it is obviously important to have factors in prognosis to delineate the 40% for whom treatment will be required. It has been accepted for many years that there are a number of factors which the clinician may find of value in his assessment of an individual case. These may be subdivided into short-term and longterm factors (Tables 7.1 and 7.2).

Short-term factors

Age and sex

It is accepted that the younger the age of onset of the disease the better the prognosis with boys having a more favourable prognosis than girls. The explanation for this seems to be that younger children are less likely to damage their epiphysis and have longer to remodel their femoral heads after healing of the disease. The unfavourable prognosis for girls is due to the fact that they have a more serious form of the disease (see 'group' below).

The stage of the disease at diagnosis

It is accepted that the earlier in the disease process the treatment is started the better the prognosis as less deformity has potentially occurred. It must also be stated that once healing is established radiologically there will be no further deterioration in the shape of the femoral head (Westin & Thompson 1977). Treatment is only indicated at this stage of the disease if it can be shown to improve congruity of the femoral head. This must be demonstrated by arthrography.

Table 7.1 Short-term prognosis.

1	Age and sex
2	The stage of the disease at diagnosis
3	Group
4	Signs of the 'head at risk'

Group

The prognosis for an individual case is proportional to the degree of radiological involvement of the epiphysis and on this basis four groups have been defined (Catterall 1971). These groups correspond to the extent of infarction present within the epiphysis (Catterall 1982). The radiological signs used in the definition of group are set out in Tabes 7.3 and 7.4, but good quality radiographs are required for their interpretation. The subchondral fracture line (Fig. 7.6) initially described by Waldenstrom (1938) and later by Caffey (1968) has recently been investigated by Salter and Thompson (1980) and is undoubtedly a very helpful sign in the assessment of group but unfortunately is only present in some 25% of cases. In untreated cases (Table 7.5) it will be seen that 90% of the good results are in Groups I and II and 90% of the poor results are in Groups III and IV.

Table 7.2 Longterm prognosis.

Favourable
Age at time of Healing
Unfavourable
Persistent lateral uncovering of the femoral head
An irregular femoral head
Premature closure to the growth plate

The signs 'at risk'

These are the clinical and radiological signs of progressive deformity of the femoral head at a stage when it is in cartilage and therefore correctable by treatment (Table 7.6) (Fig. 7.4). The presence of two or more radiological signs, particularly when associated with progressive loss of movement, is an absolute indication for treatment.

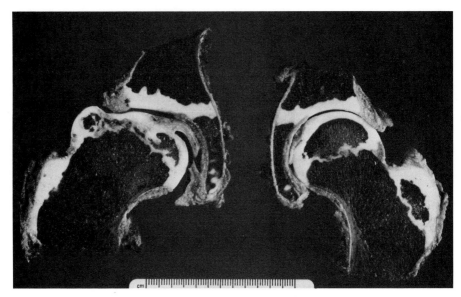

Fig. 7.3 The 'roller bearing joint'. The transverse section of the central point of the femoral head and corresponding acetabulum of a late case of Perthes disease compared with the opposite uninvolved side. The flattening produces movement of the hip in the flexion/extension axis only. Because of the varus deformity in the femoral neck the leg lies adducted and therefore short when the hip is extended and abducted when the hip is flexed.

Table 7.3 Epiphyseal signs.

Radiological signs	Group I	Group II	Group III	Group IV
Sclerosis	No	Yes	Yes	Yes
Subchondral fracture line	No	Anterior half	Posterior half	Complete
Junction involved/uninvolved segments	Clear	Clear Often 'V'	Sclerotic	No
Viable bone on growth plate	Anterior margin	Anterior half	Posterior half	No
Posterior remodelling	No	No	No	Yes
Triangular appearance to medial/lateral aspects	No	No	Occasional	Yes

Table 7.4 Metaphyseal signs.

Radiological signs	Group I	Group II	Group III	Group IV
Localized	No	Anterior	Anterior	Anterior or central
Diffuse	No	No	Yes	Yes

Table 7.5 Results of untreated cases.

	Good	Fair	Poor
Group I	27 ⎫	1	0
Group II	25 ⎭ 92%	6	2
Group III	4	7	11 ⎫
Group IV	0	4	10 ⎭ 91%
Total	54 (57%)	18 (19%)	23 (24%)

Table 7.6 Signs of the 'head at risk'.

Clinical	Progressive loss of movement
	Adduction contracture
	The heavy child
Radiological	Gageś sign
	Calcification lateral to the epiphysis
	A diffuse mataphyseal change
	Lateral subluxation
	Horizontal growth plate

Longterm factors

The literature on the longterm prognosis is increasing but its conclusions are clear. Eighty-six per cent of patients will develop arthritis by the age of 65 years but in the majority the symptoms will not become a problem until the fifth or sixth decade. One third of cases will improve after healing of the disease although a small proportion will deteriorate so that 9% will require reconstructive surgery by the age of thirty-five. The child who is going to develop the symptoms of early arthritis has disease of late onset which results in an irregular uncovered femoral head in which there is partial arrest of the growth plate and a reduced range of movement (Stulberg 1981, Catterall 1982). In essence these are a persistence of the signs of

Table 7.7 Differential diagnosis.

Bilateral cases	Unilateral cases
Multiple epiphyseal dysplasia	Infection
Spondyloepiphyseal dysplasia	Gaucher's disease
Myxoedema	Haemophilia
	Eosinophillic granuloma
	Lymphoma

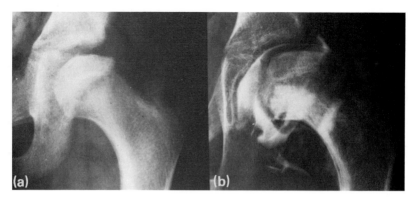

Fig. 7.4 The head 'at risk'.
(a) An anteroposterior radiograph of a child aged 7 years. There is an extensive area of sclerosis with a viable medial fragment (Group III). There is widening of the inferomedial joint space, calcification lateral to the epiphysis, and a horizontal growth plate.
(b) The arthrographic appearances confirming the subluxation and the overgrowth of the cartilagenous portion of the femoral head on its lateral aspect. The previously noted calcification lateral to the epiphysis in (a) is seen to be within the cartilagenous portion.

the 'head at risk' in the early case. In some cases however, an oval head results which, although, having femoral head deformity, shows congruity between the femoral head and the acetabulum in the neutral weightbearing position. This has been referred to as 'congruous incongruity' (Curtis 1977). In terms of these long term factors effective treatment initiated early would activate the healing process, reduce the lateral uncovering of the femoral head and restore normal movement to the hip joint without injury to the growth plate. In cases presenting late with established deformity realignment of the hip and leg to produce congruity in the neutral weightbearing position would improve the longterm outcome.

Treatment

Indications and principles of treatment

In a disease process in which 60% do well without treatment it is important to have indications for treatment so that unnecessary therapy can be avoided. In terms of the described pathology, short- and longterm factors (Tables 7.1 and 7.2), the indications and contraindications for treatment are set out in Tables 7.8 and 7.9. With an understanding of the pathology of the process of femoral head deformity, the principles of treatment would be the restoration of movement, the relief of stress through the femoral head, and the prevention of further ischaemia. Normal movement is required to prevent progressive deformity of the femoral head and to encourage remodelling of any deformity. Abduction of the leg has two effects on the hip; first to reduce the forces through the hip joint (Heikkinen *et al.* 1980) and second, to reposition the uncovered anterolateral aspect of the femoral head within the remodelling influence of the acetabulum. By doing this

Table 7.8 Indications for no treatment.

Early stage
Group I cases
Groups II, III not 'at risk'

Late stage
Cases when healing is established
Deformity of femoral head without abduction

Table 7.9 Indications for definitive treatment.

Early stage
All 'at risk' cases
Groups II, III over 7 years
Group IV cases where serious deformity has not occurred

Late stage
Hinge abduction

the abnormal forces are taken away from the lateral cartilaginous aspect of the acetabulum which resumes a more normal appearance and growth (Fig. 7.5). The cartilaginous overgrowth appears to be related to the degree of ischaemia present in the head and further episodes must therefore be prevented. When these principles are applied to the early and late stages, of the disease different methods of treatment will result. In the early stages, where the predominant pathology is cartilage overgrowth, restoration of movement with the femoral head repositioned or contained within the acetabulum would be the method of choice. In the later stages, when deformity of the femoral head has occurred and healing already established restoration of movement with the joint congruous in the neutral weightbearing position would allow the best of long term remodelling and would prevent the long term effects of hinge abduction.

Management

Early stages

It follows from these observations that the management of these children with Perthes disease presenting during the early stages will be divided into three phases:

1 diagnosis, assessment and arthrography;
2 containment of the femoral head with mobilization of the hip joint;
3 maintenance of the reduction until healing is established.

Diagnosis, assessment and arthrography

A careful history and clinical examination are important in all cases not only to exclude a Perthes-like change (Table 7.7) but also to establish the nature of its onset and the stage of the disease at presentation. These children may present with either

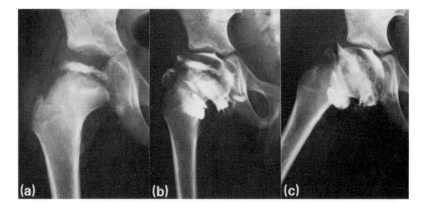

Fig. 7.5 A child aged 5 years with total involvement of the epiphysis (Group IV). There is some lateral uncovering but the shape of the acetabulum is normal.
(b) Arthrography in the neutral position shows the extent of the cartilage overgrowth and the change in overall shape both of the femoral head and the lateral aspect of the acetabulum.
(c) View in abduction showing centring of the femoral head (containment). Note the change in the shape of the lateral aspect of the acetabulum and the potential influence that this will have on remodelling.

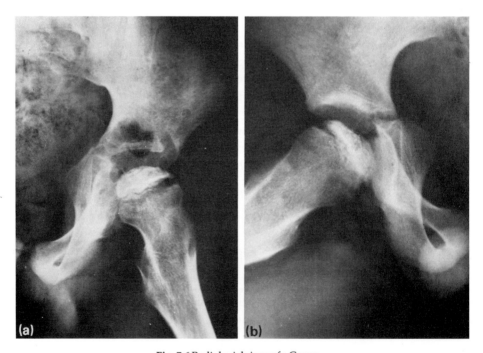

Fig. 7.6 Radiologial signs of a Group.
(a) Lateral radiograph of a Group III case. The subchondral fracture line extends into the posterior third of the epiphysis. There is extensive metaphyseal reaction.
(b) Lateral radiography of Group II case showing clear demarcation betwen involved and uninvolved segments as a 'Y' (Table 7.3).

acute symptoms in the form of 'irritable hip' or by chronic presentation with pain and limp, the symptoms of which are often truly intermittent in the early stages. In all cases clinical examination must be thorough, and include measurements of height and weight. Shortening of the involved leg is an important sign and should be looked for as the child lies down. If present it must be established whether it is due to postural adduction or due to fixed deformity in which flexion and adduction may be important components. The range of movement from the position of fixed deformity must then be noted. Limitation of abduction of the flexed hip is present in all cases at an early stage.

Radiological examination is required to exclude the differential diagnosis (Table 7.7). Radiographs also determine the stage of the disease, the group and the presence of any signs of the 'head at risk'. The most useful signs in diagnosis (Table 7.10) are widening of the inferomedial joint space, sclerosis and a subchondral

Table 7.10 Diagnosis.

Radiological signs
Widening of the inferomedial joint space
Epiphyseal sclerosis
Subchondral fracture line
A small epiphysis

Table 7.11 Principles of treatment.

Restoration and maintenance of movement
Reduction of stress through the hip joint
Prevention of further ischaemia

fracture line (Fig. 7.2a). Where there is doubt about a persisting painful hip an important diagnostic investigation is the technesium 99 polyphosphate bone scan. This investigation has been found to have an accuracy of between 95% and 98% and false positives are extremely rare (Sutherland *et al.* 1980). In many cases the diagnosis is obvious but good quality X-rays are necessary, after a period of rest, to establish the Group. They should include anteroposterior and Lauenstien views. If treatment is being considered an arthrogram is required to establish the shape of the cartilaginous part of the femoral head and the position it is best contained within the acetabulum. Arthrography is best performed under general anaesthesia and provides an ideal opportunity to reassess the hips; in particular there is the opportunity to determine whether any clinical contractures are due to fixed deformity or simple muscle spasm which is eliminated as the result of the anaesthetic. The injection may be made either through an anterior or perineal approach under the control of the image intensifier. Care must be taken not to inject too much dye as this will prevent good assessment of the shape of the femoral head. The shape of the femoral head is then determined and the best position and fit of the femoral head and acetabulum identified (Fig. 7.5). The presence of 'hinge abduction' must also be looked for and noted (Fig. 7.9b).

Containment of the femoral head, and mobilization of the hip joint

If a decision is made to proceed with definitive treatment the femoral head must be repositioned within the acetabulum to that position demonstrated by

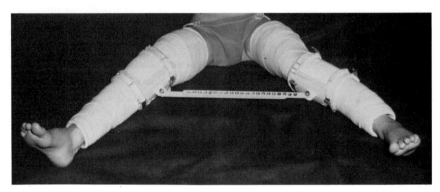

Fig. 7.7 The adjustable broomstick plaster.

arthrography and the hip joint then mobilized to restore full mobility. This is best achieved in an adjustable plaster of the broomstick type (Fig. 7.7). The position of the legs is adjusted on a daily basis progressively abducting and internally rotating the leg until the desired position has been obtained and checked radiologically. During this time the child is encouraged to move the hip as much as possible but not to stand.

Maintenance of the reduction until healing is established

It is in this aspect of treatment that the greatest controversy exists. Should therapy be conservative by splintage or radical by operation? In essence both the containment braces and femoral osteotomy achieve the same objectives and have very similar results in the young child. Most authorities would agree that bracing is an unsatisfactory method of treatment in the child over the age of seven years and that a weight removing caliper, although maintaining a good range of movement, does not seriously alter the natural history of the untreated disease. One of the questions which must be raised and answered in selective indications for treatment is whether delay will prejudice the longterm result. In the series reported by Muirhead-Allwood and Catterall (1982) delay in operation did not alter the outcome provided that operation was undertaken as soon as the 'head at risk' signs appeared. Seven out of eight cases achieved a good result and there were no poor results. The advantage of operation is that it achieves the objective treatment

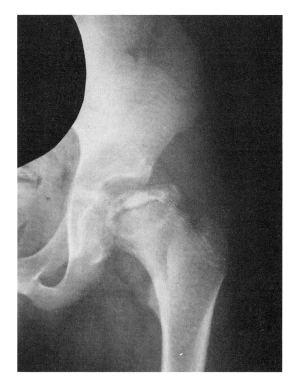

Fig. 7.8 Child aged 7 years, two years after the onset of Group III disease. There was regular pain on exercise. The involved leg was short and there was a fixed flexion/adduction contracture of the hip. The AP radiographs show marked femoral head deformity, lateral uncovering, and widening of the inferior medial joint space.

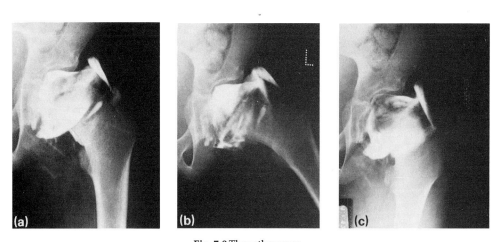

Fig. 7.9 The arthrogram.
(a) Neutral position. The lateral acetabular roof is deformed and the dye puddles medially.
(b) The appearance of hinge abduction is noted as the leg is abducted.
(c) The congruous position of the hip is in flexion and adduction.

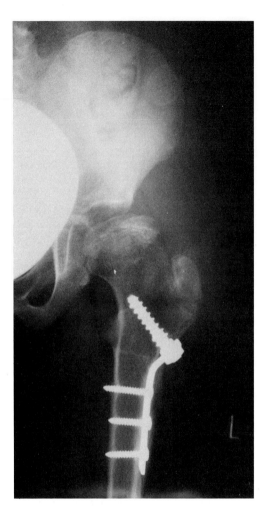

Fig. 7.10 AP radiograph taken two and a half years after abduction/extension femoral osteotomy. Note the improvement in femoral head shape and the narrowing of the inferomedial joint space.

(Lloyd-Roberts *et al.* 1976, Canario *et al.* 1980, Axer *et al.* Muirhead-Allwood & Catterall 1982), is of short duration and particularly in the older child will shorten the duration of disease by triggering the healing process. In addition there are none of the social problems of the 'child in a brace' with serious problems at school and restriction of his usual activities.

Late presentation

Children who present in the later stages of the disease may or may not have serious femoral head deformity. When leg lengths are equal and there is only slight restriction of movement it is unlikely that there is any serious deformity of the femoral head. Persisting pain during the healing stages is always a worrying symptom, particularly if there is shortening of the involved leg with fixed deformity.

An arthrogram is indicated and will commonly demonstrate 'hinge abduction' (Fig. 7.9). This arthrogram will also demonstrate the congruent position for the femoral head. Treatment is by an abduction/extension osteotomy of the femur to realign the congruent position of the hip to the neutral weightbearing position (Figs. 7.8, 7.9 and 7.10). By reversing the process of hinging this operation relieves pain and corrects leg length (Quain & Catterall 1986).

Conclusions

Much remains to be learnt about this condition whose aetiology has remained unexplained for more than 70 years. Recent investigations have identified 'the susceptible child' and this has provided an avenue of interesting investigation. With a better understanding of the pathology and natural history it is now possible to be more selective in treatment but in the older child the results of the present regimes of treatment do not provide a cause for optimism and other methods of treatment will have to be introduced for these difficult cases.

References

Axer A., Gershuni D. H., Hendel D. & Miroyski Y. (1980) Indications for femoral osteotomy in Legg–Calve–Perthes disease. *Clinical Orthopaedics and Related Research,* **150,** 78–87.

Burwell R. G., Dangerfield P. H., Hall D. J., Vernon C. L. & Harrison M. H. M. (1978) Perthes disease. An anthropometric study revealing impaired and disproportionate growth. *Journal of Bone and Joint Surgery,* **60B,** 461–77.

Caffey J. (1968) The early roentgenographic changes in essential cox vara: their significance in pathogenesis. *American Journal of Roentgenology,* **103,** 620–34.

Canario A. T., Williams L., Wientroub S., Catterall. A. & Lloyd-Roberts G. C. (1980) A controlled study of the results of femoral osteotomy in severe Perthes disease. *Journal of Bone and Joint Surgery,* **62B,** 438–40.

Catterall A. (1971) The natural history of Perthes disease. *Journal of Bone and Joint Surgery,* **53B,** 37–53.

Catterall A. (1982) Perthes disease. Is the epiphysial infarction complete? *Journal of Bone and Joint Surgery,* **64B,** 276–81.

Curtis B. H. (1977) A method for assessing outcome in Legg–Calve–Perthes syndrome. *First International Symposium in Legg–Calve–Perthes Sydrome,* Los Angeles.

Hall A. J., Barker D. J. P., Dangerfield P. H. & Taylor J. F. (1983) Perthes disease in Liverpool. *British Medical Journal,* **287,** 1757.

Harrison M. H. M., Turner M. H. & Jacobs P. (1976) Skeletal immaturity in Perthes disease. *Journal of Bone and Joint Surgery,* **58B,** 37–40.

Heikkinen E. & Puranen J. (1980) Evaluation of femoral osteotomy in the treatment of Legg–Calve–Perthes disease. *Clinial Orthopaedics and Related Research,* **150,** 60–8.

Inoue A., Freeman M. A. R., Vernon-Roberts B. & Mizuno S. (1976) The pathogenesis of Perthes disease. *Journal of Bone and Joint Surgery,* **58B,** 453–61.

Lloyd-Roberts G. C., Catterall A. & Salamon P. B. (1976) A controlled study of the indications and results of femoral osteotomy in Perthes disease. *Journal of Bone and Joint Surgery,* **58B,** 31–6.

McKibbin B. & Ralis Z. (1974) Changes found in a case of Perthes disease at necropsy. A case report. *Journal of Bone and Joint Surgery,* **56B,** 438–47.

Muirhead-Allwood W. & Catterall A. (1982) The treatment of Perthes disease. *Journal of Bone and Joint Surgery,* **64B,** 269–76.

Quain S. & Catterall A. (1986) Hinge abduction, its diagnosis and management. *Journal of Bone and Joint Surgery,* (in press).

Ralston E. L. (1955) Legg-Perthes disease and physical development. *Journal of Bone and Joint Surgery,* **37A,** 647.

Salter R. B. & Thompson G. H. (1980) Legg–Calve–Perthes disease. The prognostic significance of the subchondral fracture. Paper presented to the American Academy of Orthopaedic Surgeons 1980.

Sutherland A. D., Savage J. P., Paterson D. C. & Foster B. K. (1980) The nuclide bone scan in diagnosis and management of Perthes disease. *Journal of Bone and Joint Surgery,* **62B,** 300–6.

Stulberg S. D., Cooperman R. D. & Wallensten R. (1981) The natural history of Legg–Calve–Perthes disease. *Journal of Bone and Joint Surgery,* **63A,** 1095–108.

Waldenstrom H. (1938) The first stages of coxa plana. *Journal of Bone and Joint Surgery,* **20,** 559–66.

Westin G. & Thompson G. H. (1977) Legg–Calve–Perthes disease. The results of discontinuing treatment in reformative phase. *First Internatioal Symposium Legg–Calve–Perthes sydrome.*

Wynne-Davies R. & Gormley J. (1978) The aetiology of Perthes disease. *Journal of Bone and Joint Surgery,* **60B,** 6–14.

8

Slipped Capital Femoral Epiphysis

I. G. STOTHER

Although uncommon, slipping of the capital femoral epiphysis has been recognized for many years, Durbin (1960) attributing the first description to Ambrose Pare in 1572. The exact incidence varies throughout the world. In western Europe similar figures have been reported from Scotland with an annual occurence of 8.3 cases per 100,000 population between the ages of 11 and 16 years (Rennie 1982) and Sweden with 2–13 cases per year per 100,000 population between the ages of 7 and 16 years (Henrikson 1969). In Japan, however, the condition appears to be less common with a reported incidence of only 0.2–0.3 cases per 100,000 population between the ages of 10 and 14 (Ninomiya *et al.* 1976). Similar racial differences have been reported from North America where it would appear that the condition is commoner in the Negro population (Kelsey 1974).

Males are more commonly affected than females, the ratio ranging from 1.3:1 to 5.8:1 (Knight *et al.* 1987, Durbin 1960, Ninomiya *et al.* 1976, Wilson *et al.* 1965). Bilateral involvement is not infrequent, varying from 23% to 34% (Durbin 1960, Burrows 1957, Orofino *et al.* 1960, Wilson *et al.* 1965). Such bilateral involvement may occur simultaneously or the second slip may occur later than the first, indeed at any time until closure of the epiphyseal plate. In many cases involvement of the second side is asymptomatic so that serial radiographs should be performed until the epiphysis has fused. The majority of cases occur in patients between the ages of ten and sixteen years. Burrows (1957) reported that whereas the majority of girls presented between the ages of 11 and 13 years, most boys were slightly older, that is between 14 and 16 years at the time of diagnosis. Similar findings have been reported from Glasgow where girls were diagnosed on average at 12.2 years and boys at 13.2 years (Knight *et al.* 1987).

Aetiology

The aetiology of the condition is not clearly understood. Nevertheless, certain groups 'at risk' can be identified. Two broad categories can be defined: those in whom the stress on the epiphyseal plate is increased and those in whom strength of the epiphyseal plate is reduced.

Obesity

Obesity may increase the load on the capital epiphysis. Certainly almost half of the patients suffering from the condition have been found to be overweight (Burrows 1957). Chung *et al.* (1976) believe that, in such obese children, the loads across the epiphyseal plate complex can be high enough to cause slipping in a normal hip.

Familial susceptibility

Whilst the mode of inheritance remains uncertain, there would appear to be a materially increased chance of a second case arising in a family where a girl is already affected (Rennie 1982).

Hormonal factors

Growth hormones, sex hormones and thyroid hormones are all active at the growth plate. Harris (1950) has hypothesized that endocrine imbalance occurring during the adolescent growth spurt may be a contributory factor. Certainly the condition has its peak incidence at the time of the adolescent growth spurt. As the spurt occurs earlier in girls than in boys, this would explain the earlier presentation of the condition in females.

Whilst slipped capital femoral epiphysis is undoubtedly associated with abnormalities of pituitary and thyroid function (Heatley *et al.* 1976) it must be emphasized that it is only in a tiny minority of cases that any clinically treatable endocrine abnormality can be demonstrated. Indeed Puri *et al.* (1983) recommended that only those children who are short or obese should be screened for hypothyroidism.

Metabolic factors

Irradiation of the pelvis for childhood malignancies increases the risk of a later slip of the capital epiphysis (Chapman *et al.* 1980). The high cell turnover in the physis is thought to make it particularly susceptible to the effects of irradiation.

Pathology

In almost all cases the femoral head is displaced downwards and backwards with respect to the femoral neck. This produces an apparent varus tilt. The head remains within the acetabulum.

Morphologically, there appears to be accelerated chondrocyte death and a decrease in the amount of collagen in the matrix of the abnormal epiphysis (Agamonolis *et al.* 1985). The mechanism responsible for the changes is not clear.

Chronic synovitis has long been recognized as an invariable accompaniment of the disorder. Recently immune complexes have been found in association with this (Morrisey *et al.* 1983) and their presence supports the suggestion that slipping of the capital femoral epiphysis may have an autoimmune basis. Elevated immunoglobulins have also been identified in patients' serum (Eisenstein & Rothschild 1976) but it is unclear whether these represent a response to an antigen released in the process of slipping or whether the slipping is part of an autoimmune state.

The natural history and clinical features of slipped capital femoral epiphysis

It is convenient to consider the natural history of the condition in the following stages:

1 Stage of slipping
     (a) acute
     (b) chronic
     (c) acute on chronic
2 Stage of healing
3 Stage of complications
     (a) further slip
     (b) chondrolysis
     (c) avascular necrosis
4 Residual stage

1 Stage of slipping

The slip may occur in one of several ways. It is customary to consider slips to be acute, chronic or acute on chronic.

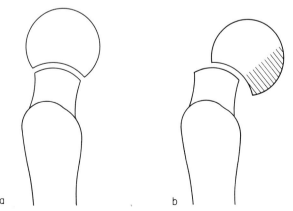

Fig. 8.1 (a) Normal lateral view of the neck and epiphysis.
(b) Acute slip of the epiphysis. The shaded area shows the posterior overhang. There is no remodelling of the neck.

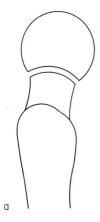

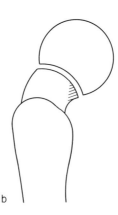

Fig. 8.2 To show chronic slip of
the epiphysis.
(a) Normal lateral.
(b) Chronic slip of epiphysis: the
shaded area shows the
buttressing of the neck with new
bone which lies under the
posterior margin of the head.
There is no posterior overhang.

a   b

An acute slip is one which occurs in a previously normal hip. A chronic slip is
one in which there has been a history of pain and limping for several weeks or
months, without there being any acute episode of more severe symptoms. In
contrast, an acute on chronic slip is one where an episode of acute, more severe
symptoms occurs in a child who has had preceding history of pain and limp.

The history, however, is only an approximate guide to the type of slip. Much
more accurate are two radiological changes seen in a lateral view of the hip. These
changes are shown diagramatically in Figs. 8.1, 8.2 and 8.3. In an acute slip, there
is no remodelling of the neck and the capital epiphysis is displaced posteriorly so
that it overhangs the back of the normal neck (Fig. 8.1). In a chronic slip, the
epiphysis has slipped but the neck has remodelled so that a buttress of new bone
lies under the epiphysis which, in consequence, does not overhang the posterior
aspect of the neck (Fig. 8.2). In an acute on chronic slip, the neck has remodelled
but the epiphysis has displaced further in the secondary acute episode and
overhangs the remodelled neck. (Fig. 8.3).

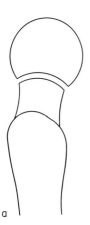

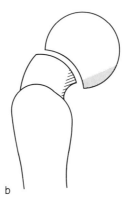

Fig. 8.3 To show acute on chronic
slip.
(a) Normal lateral.
(b) Acute on chronic slip. There is
remodelling of the neck with
posterior buttressing shown
hatched. In addition there is
posterior overhang of the
remodelled neck by the dotted
area of the epiphysis.

a   b

1(a)   Acute slipping

This is characterized by inability to walk after sustaining a major injury. Such injuries are rare and this category accounts for only a small minority of patients (Dunn 1964, Ratliffe 1968). Ratliffe (1968) has suggested that such acute traumatic slipping of the epiphysis constitutes a separate entity and is quite separate from the other forms. Perhaps this should be recognized by renaming the condition a transepiphyseal fracture. Certainly its clinical presentation is that of an acute severe injury warranting immediate hospital admission. The radiological features are those of separation at the epiphyseal plate. The capital epiphysis remains within the acetabulum. If the displacement is minimal, the epiphyseal line is widened, most noticeably in the lateral view. With increasing displacement, the neck of the femur is displaced forwards relative to the head.

These injuries should be treated like any other major epiphyseal slip by early reduction and immobilization in the reduced position (*see* Treatment). Even with expeditious treatment complications are common. These include avascular necrosis and premature fusion of the epiphyseal plate leading to shortening of the femoral neck. The frequency of these complications is a reflection of the severe trauma necessary to produce this injury.

1(b)   Chronic slipping

This is the commonest type (Burrows 1957). Displacement at presentation varies from a minimal amount to complete although the latter is very rare in the absence of surgical intervention (Howarth 1957). In a Glasgow series of 102 hips (Knight *et al.* 1987) 50% of cases had a slip of less than one-third of the diameter of the femoral neck. The slipping often seemed to occur gradually and intermittently, allowing new bone to fill the posterolateral angle between the epiphysis and the neck. This tends to stabilize the neck as well as making attempts at closed reduction both difficult and hazardous.

Clinically, patients with chronic slipping of the epiphysis present with a history of pain and limp. The two symptoms are commonly of gradual onset and initially intermittent, in the early stages only occurring after exercise. Pain is most commonly felt in the region of the hip and over the anterior aspect of the thigh. Whilst knee pain may occur as the only site of discomfort, it more often accompanies hip pain, this being the case in 37% of the Glasgow series (Knight *et al.* 1987). All patients have a limp. If there is active slipping the child will also have a Trendelenberg gait. This may not be the case if the slipping has occurred some time previously. The limp then arises as a consequence of the resulting short leg and external rotation deformity on the affected side.

Examination should be performed in the normal way with the patient lying on a couch with the pelvis immobilized. If examination takes place during the acute phase there will be concentric limitation of movement of the hip in all directions as a consequence of the associated synovitis, although the limitation resulting from the deformity will be most marked. If the slip has temporarily stabilized then the limitation of motion due to deformity is characteristically:

(a)   Loss of internal rotation.
(b)   Inability to flex the hip whilst maintaining neutral rotation. Flexion of the hip is accompanied by external rotation and abduction at the joint (Fig. 8.4).
(c)   Loss of abduction.

Other signs occur but are less common, less specific and more difficult to detect. Wasting of the thigh muscles occurs but may not be obvious, particularly in obese patients. Shortening of the affected limb is common but normally amounts to only 1–2 cm (Fig. 8.5).

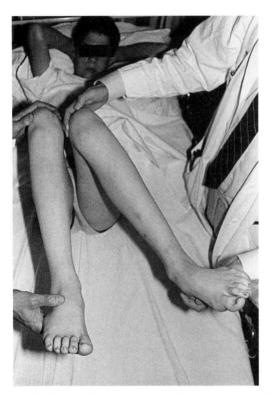

Fig. 8.4 Slipping of the right capital femoral epiphysis. The hips are flexed to a right angle, and an atttempt is being made to internally rotate both hips. The right hip lies in external rotation, the left hip can be internally rotated. (The knees are bent to about 130° for ease of photography.)

Radiographs are essential to make the diagnosis. Until two views, that is an anteroposterior and frog lateral, have been taken, the condition has not been excluded. In view of the high frequency of bilateral involvement such X-rays should always include the apparently normal side. Where the amount of slip is small and the patient is seen early in the natural history of the condition, the anteroposterior X-ray may be almost normal. Such slips are more easily seen in the lateral film which will show posterior displacement of the capital epiphysis in the neck (Fig. 8.6). Early signs in the anteroposterior view include widening of the epiphyseal

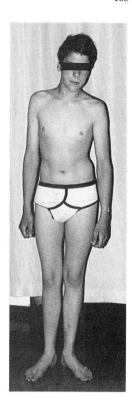

Fig. 8.5 This patient has slipping of the right capital femoral epiphysis. Note the shortening of the right leg with elevation of the left iliac crest. The right hip is held in external rotation as shown by the postion of the right patella. There is slight wasting of the right thigh.

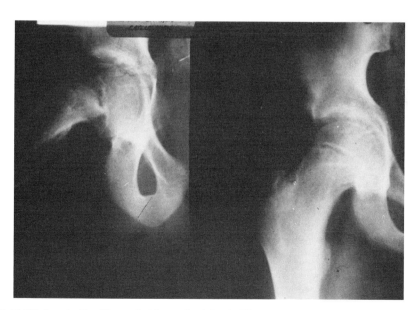

Fig. 8.6 Mild chronic slip of the capital femoral epiphysis. The anteroposterior view on the right looks almost normal. The lateral view on the left shows the curved neck with the posterior placement of the epiphysis.

line, irregularity on the neck side of the line and the head sitting low in the neck. This last sign can be highlighted by drawing a line along the superior margin of the neck. This line does not pass through the epiphysis to the same extent as on the normal side (Figs. 8.7 and 8.8). Where the slipping has occurred over several months then remodelling of the femoral neck will have taken place. By definition, such remodelling will be present in all cases of chronic slipping. The inferior border of the neck becomes curved where new bone fills in the corner between the neck and the epiphysis. Additionally, whilst the anterior aspect of the neck remodels, there is often an anterior bony knob (Fig. 8.9). The appearance of such changes is almost certainly a contraindication to attempted closed reduction.

The extent of the slip is described with reference to the radiographs. In the simplest descriptions only true displacement seen in the frog lateral view is described. Either the extent of the slip is described as a proportion of the diameter of the neck or the angular deformity between the base of the capital femoral epiphysis and the axis of the femoral shaft is described as shown in Fig. 8.10. This angular deformity can only be calculated if the angle between the base of the epiphysis and the femoral shaft on the normal side is known. The normal value is around 10°. Using the angular system of measurement, the displacement can also be calculated in the anteroposterior view as shown in Fig. 8.11. The normal

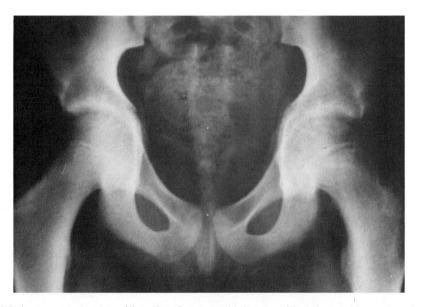

Fig. 8.7. Anteroposterior view of the pelvis showing mild slipping of the left capital femoral epiphysis. Note the low position of the head on the neck, the widening of the epiphyseal line and the irriegularity on the neck side of the line. (Compare with Figs. 8.8 and 8.9).

Fig. 8.8 Tracing of the radiograph shown in Fig. 8.7. The lines L–L and R–R are drawn along the superior border of the femoral neck. R–R on the normal side transects a segment of epiphysis, but L–L, on the slipped side does not transect the epiphysis. Line 1 points to the epiphyseal widening. Line 2 points to the irregularity on the neck side of the epiphysis.

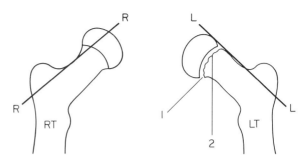

value for the angle between the base of the epiphysis and the femoral shaft in this projection is about 145°. The angular deformity is, of course, the difference between the normal and affected sides.

All these measurements are dependent upon the position of the hip when the radiographs are taken and are therefore approximate. As an alternative therefore, the slip can be categorized more simply as mild, moderate or severe. A mild slip is one where the displacement of the head is less than one-third the diameter of the femoral neck (about 30°) in the lateral view. A moderate slip is where the displacement is between one-third and one-half the diameter (between 30° and 60°) and a severe one is when it is greater than one-half.

1(c)   Acute on chronic slipping

This category includes those patients who sustain further acute displacement of

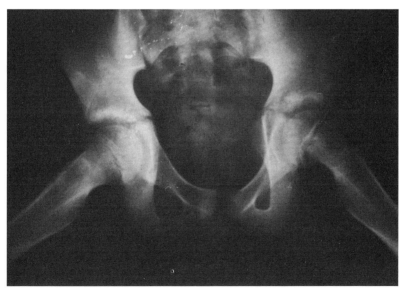

Fig. 8.9 This shows mild chronic slipping of the left capital epiphysis with posterior buttressing and an anterior knob or beak. Same case as Fig. 8.7. The slip is much more obvious in the lateral view.

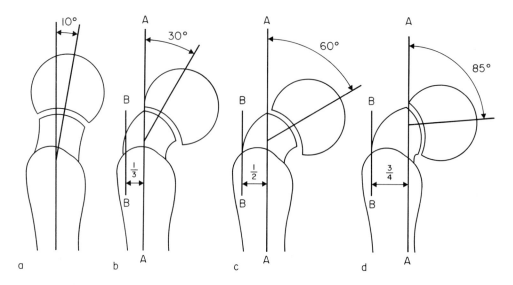

Fig. 8.10 Diagram of the lateral X-ray showing increasing amounts of epiphyseal slip.

a) No slip.

b) Mild slip.
AB; 1/3 diamater.
Neck/shaft angle
of 30°.

c) Moderate slip.
AB: 1/2 diameter.
Neck/shaft angle
of 60°.

d) Severe slip.
AB: 3/4 diameter.
Neck/shaft angle
of 85°.

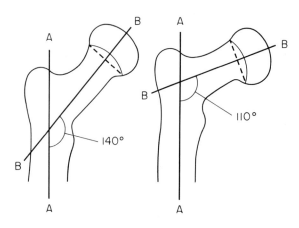

Normal   Slipped

Fig. 8.11 Anteroposterior views of
normal hip and hip with
epiphyseal slip.
AA is the axis of the femoral shaft.
BB is perpendicular to a line
drawn across the base of the
epiphysis.

the epiphysis in the presence of a persisting chronic slip.

Clinically such children have usually had minor symptoms for some months. Then, often during some sporting or athletic activity, they develop increased pain and limp on the affected side. The pain may not be very dramatic and it may be some days before the patient seeks medical advice. Findings on examination are the same as those associated with a chronic slip with the exception that restriction of movement is likely to be more severe.

Radiographs will show evidence of a longstanding slip with remodelling of the femoral neck forming a posterior break. The epiphysis, however, will overhang the bony beak. This displacement represents the extent of the acute slip (Fig. 8.12).

Following further slipping, there is likely to be considerable irritability of the hip. This will settle with a few days' bedrest in skin traction. Whilst attempted

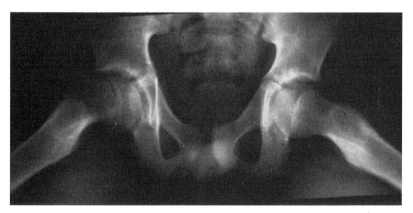

Fig. 8.12 Frog lateral view showing acute on chronic slip of the left capital epiphysis. The epiphysis overhangs the remodelled neck posteriorly.

reduction of the acute component of the slip has been advocated, the value of such manoeuvres is controversial and is not without risk to the blood supply to the epiphysis (Howarth 1957).

2   The stage of healing

A slipped epiphysis is potentially unstable. Once slipping has occurred, further displacement may take place with only minimal symptoms. Additionally, further episodes of acute slip may be precipitated by normal or more particularly, athletic activities. This risk disappears only when healing is complete, that is when the epiphyseal plate has fused.

When chronic slipping has occurred remodelling of the femoral neck takes place. New bone is added inferoposteriorly, this acting as a buttress stabilizing the epiphysis in its new position. At the same time a 'beak' of the femoral neck is exposed anterosuperiorly. This may impinge against the acetabulum and cause limitation of abuction and internal rotation. If the epiphysis stabilizes, remodelling takes place so that the range of motion of the hip may increase for several years, even after closure of the epiphyseal plate (O'Brien & Fahey 1977) (Fig. 8.21).

3   Stage of complications

Here are included those complications that may arise between the time of diagnosis and closure of the epiphyseal plate.

3(a) Further slipping

Further slip may occur if the condition is not treated. This view is supported by the fact that the average duration of symptoms has been found to be shorter in patients with slight slipping compared to those with severe (Jacobs 1972, Wilson *et al.* 1965). Slipping of the opposite femoral epiphysis occurs in about one-quarter of all cases. The extent of this slip bears no relationship to the extent of the slip on the first affected side. The time between the slip occuring in one side and the other is also variable. Only occasionally do the two appear to be affected simultaneously. The time lapse may be as much as 4 years. Treatment designed to prevent progressive slipping may be ineffective. For example, the epiphysis may 'grow off' pins inserted to stabilize it (Fig. 8.13). Similarly, grafts inserted across the physis may not fuse. For these reasons, it is of great importance that, whatever procedure has been undertaken, radiographic follow-up should continue until fusion of the growth plate has occurred.

3(b) Chondrolysis

Chondrolysis may be defined as a rapidly progressive narrowing of the joint space, accompanied by stiffness, secondary to loss of articular cartilage in the hip joint (Fig. 8.14). Such changes may involve either the whole joint space or be limited to the superior weightbearing part. It can occur whatever line of treatment is followed whether this be simple relief of weightbearing, cast immobilization or any of the various forms of surgery.

The loss of articular cartilage occurs on both the femoral and acetabular surfaces. Histology shows variable destruction of the articular surfaces and their replacement with fibrocartilage. Lymphoid infiltration of the synovium and fibrosis and thickening of the capsule are additional findings. The cause of these changes is not clear. Penetration of the joint by pins inserted in attempts at surgical stabilization has been suggested as a possible cause (Bishop *et al.* 1978) but others have found no such relationship (Bennet *et al.* 1984). Obviously this cannot be a factor in those cases which occur without surgical intervention. As the changes occur in both sides of the joint, a vascular aetiology is unlikely. The synovial changes suggests that the condition may have an autoimmune rather than a mechanical or vascular basis.

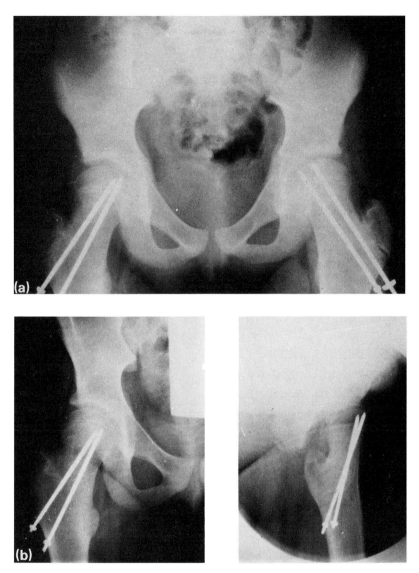

Fig. 8.13 (a) Shows the hips shortly after pinning.
(b) Shows how the epiphysis has grown clear of the pins.

Negroes are more likely to develop this complication (Orofino *et al.* 1960). Notwithstanding, it should be suspected in any patient in whom the range of movement does not progressively improve during the immediate postoperative period. The resulting stiffness is occasionally accompanied by pain. Sometimes the symptoms do not manifest themselves until considerably later, perhaps up to six months after the epiphysis has been stabilized.

Radiology shows a reduction in the normal joint space (4mm–5mm) of at least

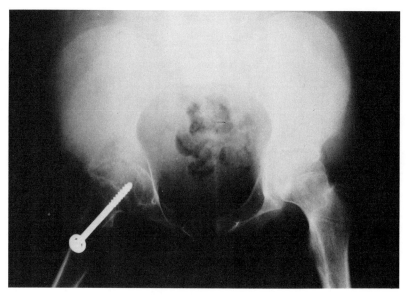

Fig. 8.14 The right slipped epiphysis has been screwed *in situ*. There is acute chondrolysis with loss of joint space on this side.

25%. Periarticular osteoporosis and erosions of subcortical bone are additional features (Goldman *et al.* 1978). Whilst the osteoporosis might be ascribed to the disease, the erosions, particularly following a surgical procedure, may well suggest infection. The white cell count and ESR, however, are normal.

Treatment is essentially symptomatic. When the pain is severe, analgesics and traction are indicated. Once the acute phase is over then the patient can be mobilized, nonweightbearing, under the supervision of a physiotherapist. Jacobs (1972) suggests manipulation under anaesthesia as a means of obtaining an increased range of movement once the pain has settled.

The residual disability is very variable and depends upon the extent of the cartilage necrosis. Some patients go onto ankylose. Others develop osteoarthrosis over a period of a few years. Definitive treatment, for example arthrodesis, should be postponed for at least 2 years after the onset of symptoms as some improvement may occur during this time. Around half the patients who develop acute cartilage necrosis will be severely disabled as a result (Wilson *et al.* 1965, Gage *et al.* 1978).

3(c) Acute avascular necrosis

Avascular necrosis does not occur in the untreated hip (Howarth 1957). Interference with the blood supply, particularly with the posteroinferior retinacular vessels, as a result of operative intervention, is the basic cause. Depending upon the extent of the vascular injury either the whole, or only part, of the capital epiphysis may be involved (Fig. 8.15).

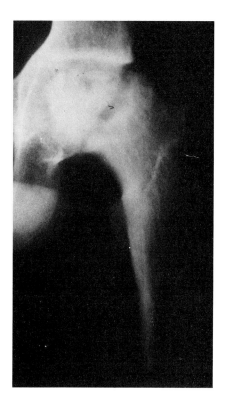

Fig. 8.15 Acute avascular necrosis with segmental collapse. The hip had been pinned *in situ*.

High cervical osteotomy is the procedure most likely to produce this complication (Gage *et al.* 1978), when incidence may be as high as 28%. Not all authors, however, report such a formidable rate. Thus, Dunn and Angel (1978) reported only two cases of avascular necrosis in 23 hips treated by high cervical osteotomy for moderate or severe slip. Similarly, Fish (1984) had only one case in a series of 42 osteotomies. It must be emphasized, however, that most reported series of this procedure record a high incidence of avascular necrosis and this remains the main reason for the reluctance of many surgeons to perform it.

The features of avascular necrosis may not develop for up to 18 months after surgery. Then, pain and stiffness are the cardinal clinical features. Radiologically, sclerosis, fragmentation and collapse of the epiphysis are characteristic.

To a large extent, treatment is symptomatic. The initial symptoms can normally be dealt with by a period of bedrest and traction followed by gradual mobilization, initially nonweightbearing in crutches. If collapse of the head exposes the acetabular joint surface to erosion by metallic internal fixation devices, these should be removed. Maintenance of congruity should be attempted by treatment along the lines of that usually advised for Perthes disease. The residual functional deficit depends upon the extent of the involvement of the head as well as the degree of collapse of the capital epiphysis. Early degenerative changes are a common sequela.

4   Residual disability

It is difficult to know the natural history of untreated slipping of the capital femoral epiphysis. If progressive slipping occurs, the end result is likely to be shortening, in extreme cases of up to 5 cm (Boyer *et al.* 1981), an external rotation deformity and a limp. Only a very few will be unlucky enough to suffer the complications of acute avasuclar necrosis or chondrolysis with the resultant development of severe arthritic changes within the joint and even those with unreduced moderate slips are likely to have remarkably little trouble (Howarth 1957, Wilson *et al.* 1965, O'Brien & Fahey 1977). It is against this background that the indications for surgery must be considered. Without surgery the complications of anaesthesia, infection and avasular necrosis are avoided and those of chondrolysis greatly reduced. These complications are kept to a minimum if pinning or bone-pegging *in situ* is performed. The risks are increased when basal or intertrochanteric osteotomy is performed and are maximal after open reduction and high cervical osteotomy. Whatever line of treatment is embarked upon it is of the utmost importance that the advantages, both short- and longterm, outweigh the risks for the individual patient. If doubt exists it is better not to operate.

The treatment of slipped capital femoral epiphysis

The aim of treatment is to secure as normal a hip as possible with the maximum range of movement, no pain and the least risk of the late development of degenerative changes. Before embarking on a treatment programme, the surgeon must know:

1   the type of slip (acute, chronic or acute on chronic);
2   the degree of slip;
3   the state of the epiphyseal plate (open or closed).

The various treatment options, which can be summarized as follows, then have to be considered:

1   closed reduction and immobilization;
2   open reduction, high cervical osteotomy and internal fixation;
3   immobilization in the displaced position;
4   corrective intertrochanteric or basal osteotomy to restore the normal range of hip motion;
5   'knobectomy', excision of the anterosuperior part of the femoral neck if this obstructs motion.

Closed reduction and immobilization

Closed reduction, either by traction or manipulation under anaesthesia has a very limited place. It is, perhaps, only indicated in those rare cases of acute traumatic slip caused by severe trauma. Then, the reduction can be checked by X-ray screening and the position held either by application of a hip spica with the leg in internal rotation and abduction or by the insertion of Moore's pins (*see* p. 177). The results of attempting such manipulative reduction in cases of acute on chronic slipping are not good. Many apparently successful reductions probably represent no more than a change in the X-ray projection (Griffith 1973). Closed reduction is contraindicated in chronic slipping because of the very real risk of producing avascular necrosis.

Open reduction, high cervical osteotomy and internal fixation

This is probably the most controversial of all the methods of treatment used in this disorder. Whilst it undoubtedly offers the surgeon the best chance of restoring near normal anatomy in a hip with moderate or severe displacement of the capital femoral epiphysis, this is achieved at the risk of producing avascular necrosis. The procedure may be indicated if there is a moderate or severe chronic or acute on chronic slip, the epiphyseal plate is open and it is not technically feasible to internally fix the epiphysis in the slipped position (usually a slip of more than 60°). The choice then is to carry out open reduction, high cervical osteotomy and internal fixation or alternatively a corrective osteotomy either at the base of the neck or in the intertrochanteric region (Kramer *et al.* 1976, Southwick 1967).

The aim of open reduction and high cervical osteotomy is to anatomically reduce the femoral head and, at the same time, avoid causing changes to the posterior retinacular vessels. To achieve this, the posterior bony beak in the neck must be removed and the neck shortened slightly (Fig. 8.16).

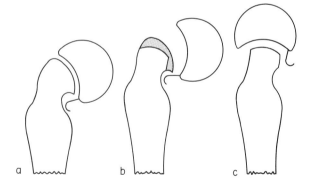

Fig. 8.16 Open reduction and high cervical osteotomy. Lateral views of hip.
(a) Pre-operative view to show posterior slip of epiphysis and posterior breaking of neck.
(b) Stippled area to be removed by osteotomy.
(c) Postosteotomy and after repositioning of epiphysis. The posterior retinacular vessels are not stretched.

Operative technique

Dunn (1969) advocates a lateral approach to the hip. The greater trochanter and the attached gluteus medius is elevated through the growth plate. The hip joint capsule is exposed and incised along its length, this incision being extended around the edge of the acetabulum. The neck is then exposed. The vascular synovium in the posterior neck is carefully elevated from the neck, at the same time maintaining its continuity with the head. The position of the growth plate is defined and is then gently freed using a wide gouge. The head retracts into the acetabulum. The neck is then osteotomized shortening it and removing the posterior neck as shown in Fig. 8.16. After scraping the remains of the growth plate from it, the head is reduced on the neck. The posterior retinaculum should be slack and, in the event of there being tension, the neck should be shortened further. The position is then held by 3 pins inserted from the lateral side of the femur. Radiographs are taken to check the reduction as well as the length of the pins. The synovium and capsule are closed and the greater trochanter reattached with a screw.

Postoperative treatment consists of 4 weeks' traction followed by mobilization, nonweightbearing on crutches, until there is radiological evidence of closure of the epiphyseal plate, usually 2–3 months postoperatively.

Fish (1984) has described an essentially similar procedure using an anterolateral approach. He exposes the neck and defines the physis with a needle. A curved wedge of bone, adjacent to the epiphyseal plate, is then removed piecemeal. The cartilage is then curretted away. By flexing abducting and internally rotating the thigh, the hip is reduced and held in place with pins. Postoperatively the patient is nursed free in bed until comfortable and then mobilized nonweightbearing on crutches until the epiphyseal plate is radiologically united.

It must be emphasized that these are not technically easy or forgiving procedures.

Immobilization in the displaced position

Where the slip is of less than half the diameter of the femoral neck and the epiphysis is still open, then immobilization in the displaced portion must be regarded as the treatment of choice. Even when the displacement is more serious, bone graft epiphysiodesis should still be considered (Boyer *et al.* 1981).

Such immobilization should be undertaken as soon as is practicable after the condition has been diagnosed. Initially bedrest and traction will reduce the associated pain and spasm and perhaps prevent or minimize further slip.

The definitive method of immobilization may be by either external measures (traction and hip spica) or internal measures (internal fixation and bone graft). Whichever method of immobilization is chosen, it should be continued until the epiphysis has fused if there is to be no risk of further slip.

External immobilization

Prolonged immobilization in a hip spica should be avoided as it is associated with residual stiffness and chondrolysis. Green (1944) however, found that a combination of traction followed by a period of up to 3 months in a hip spica with the affected hip in slight flexion and maximal internal rotation and a further spell of traction followed by physiotherapy was an effective method of treatment. Wright and King (1956) sought to avoid the risks of stiffness by using broomstick plasters holding the legs in internal rotation and abduction. These plasters allow flexion and extension as the only involvements at the hip joint.

Prolonged traction also has potential drawbacks. Skin problems and growth disturbance, particularly around the knee may occur. In view of this it is probably better to restrict traction to 6 weeks and, after that time to use some other form of immobilization. Bedrest without traction or the use of crutches does not reliably prevent further slip.

All forms of external fixation must be continued until the epiphysis has closed and this may take several months. External fixation requires cooperation by the patient and his close supervision by the surgeon. If this can be achieved the risks of complications, most notably infection and avascular necrosis, are avoided. If, however, the circumstances do not permit or external fixation fails to stabilize the epiphysis, then internal fixation is a widely practised alternative. Some would go as far as to say that all cases should be treated surgically (Carlioz *et al.* 1984).

Internal fixation in the displaced position

Early attempts at internal fixation used large diameter triangular nails. These devices were developed for use in the osteoporotic bone of the elderly and are much less suited to the hard bone of the young patient. Attempts to hammer them into the epiphysis may result in its separation at the growth plate. This increases the risk of avascular necrosis. Additionally, the large entry hole in the lateral femoral cortex predisposes to the development of a subtrochanteric fracture when the patient starts to mobilize (Wiberg 1959). For these reasons the use of such devices has been largely abandoned. The epiphysis can be much more easily rendered stable by the use of two or three small diameter pins. Alternatively bone screws may be used.

Internal fixation with Moore's pins

Small diameter pins which can be driven across the epiphysis are now widely used. The pins have a cutting point to minimize the risk of distracting the growth plate during their introduction.

Operative technique

The procedure is performed under general anaesthesia. The patient is immobilized on a fracture table and X-ray screening equipment is positioned so that anteroposterior and lateral views of the head and neck of the femur can be obtained throughout. The affected leg is placed in slight abduction and internal rotation (Fig. 8.17). A lateral approach to the upper femur is made. Using X-ray screening,

2 or 3 pins are driven (Fig. 8.18) from the lateral femoral cortex up the femoral neck and across the growth plate into the epiphysis. The position may be adjusted as necessary. Nuts are then placed in the outer ends of the pins and tightened against the lateral femoral cortex. The outer ends of the pins are then trimmed (Fig. 8.19).

Positioning of the pins may be difficult if there is much slip. It is useful to

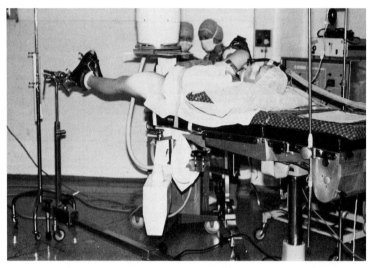

Fig. 8.17 The patient on the traction table. The left leg is in slight abduction and internal rotation. The X-ray C-arm is positioned between the patients knees with the right leg widely abducted.

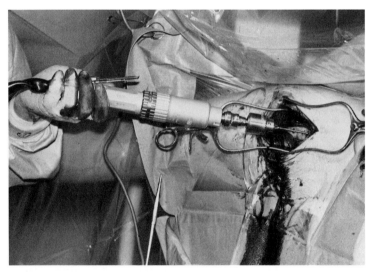

Fig. 8.18 The upper lateral femoral contex of the left leg has been exposed and a Moore's pin is being inserted with a low speed air drill. (The nut has been inserted on the pin as the drill chuck tends to damage the thread.)

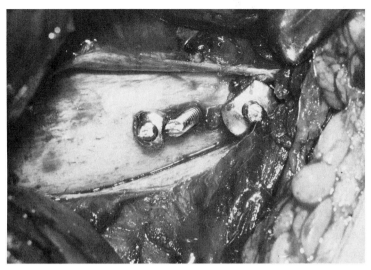

Fig. 8.19 Close up view of the lateral femoral cortex after the insertion of 3 pins and 2 nuts.

remember that the epiphysis has slipped backwards relative to the femoral neck so that access through the neck into the head can be improved if the hip is internally rotated and the pins introduced from an anterolateral rather than a true lateral position. Obesity, as is not uncommonly associated, may add to the operative difficulties.

At least two, and preferably three, pins should be inserted. To ensure stability, they must cross the physeal plate and enter the bone of the capital epiphysis. Care must be taken that the pins are not inserted too far. Even pins which may appear to lie in the capital epiphysis may in fact penetrate the joint space (Bennet *et al.* 1984). It is a wise precaution to move the joint to check there is no grating in motion before completing the operation. Any pins which are too long should be withdrawn. The ideal pin position is one of divergence although, in patients with considerable slip, this may be difficult to achieve (Fig. 8.20).

Postoperatively the patient may be nursed free in bed. Mobilization may be started 48 hours later when crutch walking, taking as much weight as is comfortable can be allowed. Most patients dispense with their crutches after about two weeks.

All patients should be followed up to check both the state of the affected hip and that on the 'normal' side. Radiographs should be taken at about 3 monthly intervals or more frequently should complications occur. Even properly inserted pins may lose their grip in the epiphysis, either because they back out or because the epiphysis grows off them. If this occurs before the epiphysis has fused then the pins should be removed and longer pins inserted in the same tracks. In thin patients, some discomfort may be felt over the outer ends of the pins. The risk of this occurence is minimized at the time of operation by cutting the pins short and ensuring that they are covered by muscle at the time of wound closure. Usually

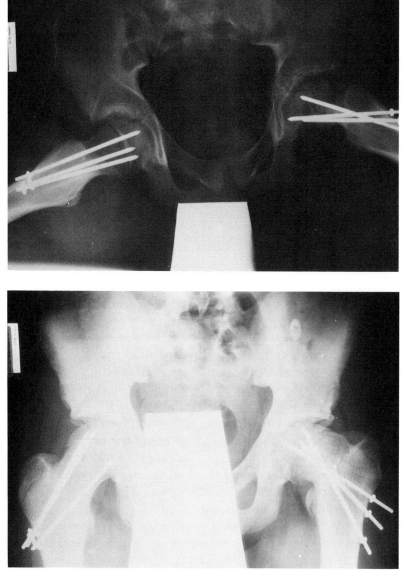

Fig. 8.20 This shows good pin placement with divergence of the pins on both the anteroposterior and lateral views although at least one pin transgresses the joint. The slip here is 60° on the lateral view.

reassurance is adequate treatment. Occasionally the nuts become undone and separate from the pins. If this occurs they should be retrieved surgically before they disappear from view. Infection is rare but in the event of its occurrence, high dosages of the appropriate antibiotic should be given. If this fails to settle the condition within a few days, then the pins should be removed. The pins should, in any case, be removed once the epiphysis has fused. Ideally, X-ray facilities should be available in case of complications. The previous incision is reopened and, as always, all the pins should be located before any of them are removed. The ends of the pins should be cleared of soft tissues and overlying tissue and the nuts unscrewed. The pins can then be loosened by holding them in a chuck and twisting them gently first one way and then the other. Once loosened they can be removed by rotating anticlockwise. If the pins are forcibly or rapidly twisted they may break. If they are jammed, a narrow gouge can be introduced alongside them to try to free them. If they break it may be necessary to window the lateral femoral cortex with either a gouge or a cannulated drill to provide access for the insertion of a heavy needle holder or similar gripping instrument. That said, it is probably wiser to leave broken pins *in situ* rather than weaken the lateral cortex by making several large holes. The presence of broken pins, however, may interfere with subsequent surgery for osteoarthritis.

Bone grafting in the displaced position

In the majority of cases, the insertion of a bone graft across the epiphyseal plate will result in its closure within 2–3 months. The procedure has the advantage that no further surgery for removal of implanted material is necessary. Excellent results have been reported (Howarth 1957, Weiner *et al.* 1984). Weiner (1984) suggests that the complications of bone graft epiphysiodesis are fewer than those of internal fixation with pins and that the serious complications of avascular necrosis and chondrolyis are less frequent.

Graft resorption and further displacement of the epiphysis are the two most commonly reported complications. Weiner (1984), however, claims that the use of a corticocancellous graft reduces the incidence of resorption and he records only one such case in 159 chronic slips treated in this way. In the same review further slip occurred in 4 patients.

Bone graft epiphysiodesis can be used to stabilize a greater degree of slip than can pin fixation as the graft passes only across the neck into the epiphysis. The procedure warrants careful consideration for the treatment of moderate or severe slipping as the complication rate is low compared to that of transcervical or intertrochanteric osteotomies and, the long term results of accepting moderate displacement are remarkably good.

Operative technique (Weiner *et al.* 1984)

Under general anaesthesia and with the patient supine on the operating table an anterior or lateral approach to the hip joint is made. The capsule is opened and the neck exposed. An anterosuperior window is cut into the femoral neck and a hollow mill drilled into the epiphysis under X-ray control. The tunnel is curetted and corticocancellous bone driven into it. The position of the graft is checked radiologically. The wound is closed in layers. If there has been an acute slip the patient is immobilized for 6 weeks in a hip spica. Otherwise they are nursed free in bed and subsequently mobilized nonweightbearing on crutches until the epiphyseal plate shows radiological evidence of closure.

Corrective basal or intertrochanteric osteotomy

When the epiphyseal slip is more than half the diameter of the femoral neck, there is often marked restriction of movement of the hip joint and the leg is held in fixed external rotation. When assessing the range of motion of the joint it is important to remember that, in the early stages, restriction of movement will be due, at least in part, to the associated synovitis. Consequently, if surgery to improve the range of motion is contemplated, it is important to treat the patient with three weeks' traction to allow the pain and spasm to settle so that the mechanically possible range of motion can be assessed.

Restricted movement at the hip combined with shortening secondary to the slip, may give the patient an ugly limp. A decision as to what form of treatment is appropriate must take into consideration the following points:

1   If the physis is still open, although open reduction and high cervical osteotomy can restore the anatomy as near to normal as is possible, it carries the highest risk of avascular necrosis.
2   If the epiphysis is still open, bone graft epiphysiodesis will stabilize the epiphysis and allow remodelling to occur. Remodelling will continue for up to two years after the epiphysis has fused. The risk of avascular necrosis after this procedure

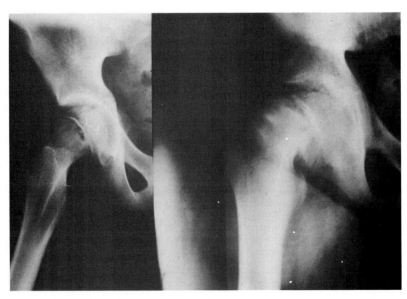

Fig. 8.21 In this case there has been a progressive untreated epiphyseal slip. Note the increase in slip between left and right and also the remodelling of the neck with loss of the superior knob.

is relatively small but the extent of correction is unpredicatable (Fig. 8.21).

3 If the epiphysis has fused then osteotomy at the base of the neck or in the intertrochanteric region reverses the deformity in the subcapital region. This procedure can also be performed whilst the plate is still open. Whilst the risk of avascular necrosis with these procedures is much lower than that associated with high cervical osteotomy, it does nevertheless occur (Salvati *et al.* 1980) as does joint space narrowing although this may be transitory.

Southwick osteotomy through the lesser trochanter

Rao *et al.* (1984) and Southwick (1967) advocate corrective osteotomy when the degree of slip is between 30° and 70° in either the anteroposterior or lateral radiograph of the hip. The change in the epiphysis–shaft angle in the anteroposterior view can be corrected by excising a wedge of bone based laterally from the intertrochanteric region of the femur as shown in Fig. 8.22. The change in the epiphysis–shaft angle in the frog lateral represents the increased retroversion of the head relative to the shaft and can be corrected by excising a wedge of bone based anteriorly (Fig. 8.23). In order to determine the wedges to be excised, radiographs in the anteroposterior and lateral planes must be available and templates should be prepared from them (Fig. 8.24). The templates should be metallic and sterilizable and can be joined together as shown. The effect of excising given sizes of wedge can be most easily assessed by taking tracings of the X-ray plates and actually cutting out the proposed wedges and aligning the remaining parts of the femur. The maximum recommended correction is 45° in the anterior plane and 60° in the lateral plane. The procedure is carried out with the patient placed on a traction table. Screening facilities should be available. A lateral approach to the upper femur is made and the bone exposed subperiosteally. Psoas is detached at the lesser trochanter. The junction of the anterior and lateral surfaces of the shaft are identified making allowance for any fixed external rotation. The junction is then marked using an osteotome so as to provide orientation. The wedges of bone to be removed are then marked out with the template in place, at the level

Fig. 8.22 Osteotomy at level of lesser trochanter. Anteroposterior view.
(a) Shows a 30° wedge based laterally. Note that the wedge does not extend right to the medial cortex of the shaft.
(b) Shows the correction of epiphysis/shaft angle achieved by excising such a wedge.

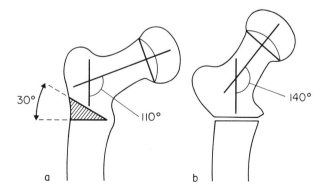

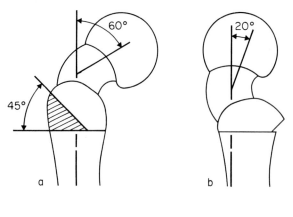

Fig. 8.23 Osteotomy at the level of the lesser trochanter, lateral view. (a) Shows a 45° wedge based anteriorly (the maximum recommended). Again the wedge does not extend completely across the shaft of the femur. (b) Shows the correction of epiphysis/shaft angle achieved by excising such a wedge.

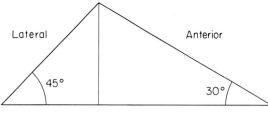

Fig. 8.24 Template prepared for case shown in Figs. 8.21 and 8.22. The actual size of template is determined from the X-rays and it is suggested that slightly smaller and slightly larger ones are also made.

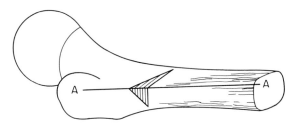

Fig. 8.25 The line AA marks the junction of the anterior and lateral surfaces of the upper femur. The wedge to be excised is outlined.

of the lesser trochanter (Fig. 8.25). The appropriate wedges of bone are then removed using an osteotome or power saw. At this stage the medial cortex is still intact. A fixation device is inserted into the proximal fragment to gain control of it. A Coventry Paediatric lag screw, a blade plate or a simple compression plate are all suitable. The transverse limb of the osteotomy is then completed through to the medial cortex.

The distal femur is then abducted, flexed and, if necessary internally rotated, the osteotomy is reduced and is held in place with the chosen plate and screws. Up to 30° of internal rotation may be necessary to allow the patella to face anteriorly.

Postoperative management depends upon the rigidity of fixation achieved. If doubt exists, a hip spica for 6–8 weeks is advisable. Otherwise the patient can be nursed free in bed for the same period and then mobilized nonweightbearing. The osteotomy usually unites by about 3 months and weightbearing can be commenced at that stage.

Variations in this basic technique have been described with osteotomies placed both in the trochanteric region (Ireland & Newman 1978) and at the base of the neck (Barmada *et al.* 1978, Kramer *et al.* 1976).

'Knobectomy'; excision of the anterosuperior part of the femoral neck

Excision of the projecting anterosuperior margin of the neck has long been advocated as a means of increasing the range of motion of the hip. Poland (1898) is usually credited with first performing this procedure. Heyman *et al.* reviewed their results in 1957. When the capital epiphysis displaces backwards the anterosuperior part of the femoral neck is exposed and may abut against the acetabular margin and in so doing, limit abduction and internal rotation and additionally, make flexion possible only if accompanied by external rotation. Excision of the projecting part of the neck may usefully increase the range of motion provided that abutment can be demonstrated. The procedure may be carried out whether or not epiphyseal fusion has occurred.

Operative technique

With the patient supine and the affected leg draped so as to allow free movement, the hip is approached anteriorly. The anterosuperior part of the joint capsule is opened longitudinally. The margin of the articular surface is identified by adducting and externally rotating the hip and is safeguarded. Flexion, abduction and internal rotation of the hip are carried out to check that impingement of the head against the acetabulum is taking place. If that is indeed the case then the bony prominence is excised using an osteotome or burr. Ideally, a concave surface is left. The range of motion is checked before closure. If the epiphyseal plate is open, an epiphysiodesis may be performed at the same time. Unless epiphysiodesis has been carried out then mobilization as symptoms allow is permitted in the post operative period.

All procedures for correcting the more severe epiphyseal slips place considerable demands on the skill of the surgeon and the patience of the adolescent patient. In view of this, if there is any doubt about the advisability of corrective surgery, then surgery should probably be deferred.

References

Agamonolis D. P., Weiner D. S. & Lloyd J. K. (1985) Slipped capital femoral epiphysis: A pathological study. *Journal of Paediatric Orthopaedics,* **5,** 47–58.

Barmada R., Bruch R. F., Gimbel J. S. & Ray R. D. (1978) Base of the neck extracapsular osteotomy for correction of deformity in SCFE. *Clinical Orthopaedics and Related Research,* **132,** 98–101.

Bennet G. C., Koreska J., & Rang M. (1984) Pin placement in slipped capital femoral epiphysis. *Journal of Paediatric Orthopaedics,* **4,** 574–8.

Bishop J. O., Oley T. J., Stephenson C. T. & Tullas H. S. (1978) Slipped capital femoral epiphysis: A study of 50 cases in black children. *Clinical Orthopaedics and Related Research,* **135,** 93–6.

Beyer D. W., Mickelson M. R. & Ponseti I. V. (1981) Slipped capital femoral epiphysis: A long term follow up of 121 patients. *Journal of Bone and Joint Surgery,* **63A,** 85–95.

Burrows J. (1957) Slipped upper femoral epiphysis: Characteristics of 100 cases *Journal of Bone and Joint Surgery,* **39B,** 641–58.

Carlioz H., Vogt J. C., Barba L., Doursounian L. (1984) Treatment of SCFE: 80 cases operated on over 10 years. *Journal of Paediatric Orthopaedics,* **4,** 153–61.

Chapman J. A., Deakin D. C. & Green J. H. (1980) Slipped upper femoral epiphysis after radiotherapy. *Journal of Bone and Joint Surgery,* **62B,** 337–9.

Chung S. M. K., Batterman S. C. & Brighton C. (1976) Shear strength of the human femoral capital epiphysis. *Journal of Bone and Joint Surgery,* **58A,** 94–103.

Dunn D. M. (1964) The treatment of adolescent slipping of the upper femoral epiphysis. *Journal of Bone and Joint Surgery,* **46B,** 621–9.

Dunn D. M. & Angel J. C. (1978) Replacement of the femoral head by open operation in severe adolescent slipping of the upper femoral epiphysis. *Journal of Bone and Joint Surgery,* **60B,** 394–403.

Durbin F. C. (1960) Treatment of slipped upper femoral epiphysis. *Journal of Bone and Joint Surgery,* **42B,** 289–302.

Eisenstein A. & Rothschild S. (1976) Biochemical abnormalities in patients with SCFE and chondrolysis. *Journal of Bone and Joint Surgery,* **58A,** 459–67.

Fish J. (1984) Cuneiform osteotomy of the femoral neck in the treatment of SCFE. *Journal of Bone and Joint Surgery,* **66A,** 1153–68.

Gage J., Sundberg A., Nolan D., Sletten R. & Winter R. (1978) Complications after cuneiform osteotomy for moderately or severely slipped capital femoral epiphysis. *Journal of Bone and Joint Surgery,* **60A,** 157–65.

Goldman A., Schneider R. & Martel W. (1978) Acute chondrolysis complicating SCFE. *American Journal of Roentgenology,* 945–50.

Green W. T. (1945) Slipping of the upper femoral epiphysis: Diagnostic and therapeutic considerations. *Archives of Surgery,* **50,** 19–33.

Griffith M. G. (1973) The morphology of slipped upper femoral epiphysis. *Journal of Bone and Joint Surgery,* **55B,** 653.

Hall J. E. (1957) The results of treatment of slipped femoral epiphysis. *Journal of Bone and Joint Surgery,* **39B,** 659–73.

Harris R. W. (1950) The endocrine basis for slipping of the upper femoral epiphysis. An experimental study. *Journal of Bone and Joint Surgery,* **32B,** 5–11.

Heatley F. W., Greenwood R. H. & Boase D. L. (1976) Slipping of UFE in patients with intracranial tumours causing hypopiuitarism and clinical compression. *Journal of Bone and Joint Surgery,* **58B,** 169–75.

Henrikson B. (1969) The incidence of slipped capital femoral epiphysis. *Acta Orthopaedica Scandinavica,* **40,** 365–72.

Heyman S., Herndon C. & Strong J. (1957) Slipped femoral epiphysis with severe displacement: A conservative operative technique. *Journal of Bone and Joint Surgery,* **39A,** 293–303.

Howorth B. (1957) Slipping of the upper femoral epiphysis. *Clinical Orthopaedics,* **10,** 148–73.

Ireland J. & Newman P. (1978) Triplane osteotomy for severely slipped upper femoral epiphysis. *Journal of Bone and Joint Surgery,* **60B,** 390–3.

Jacobs B. (1972) Chondrolysis after epiphysiosis. *American Academy of Orthopaedic Surgeons Instructional Course Lecture,* **21,** 224–6.

Kelsey J. (1974) Epidemiology of SCFE: A review. *Paediatrics,* **51,** 1042–50.

Knight D. J., Dreghorn C. & Maind S. C. (1987) Slipped capital femoral epiphysis in Glasgow. *Journal of Paediatric Orthopaedics,* **7,** 283–7.

Kramer W., Craig W. & Noels S. (1976) Compensating osteotomy at the base of the femoral neck for SCFE. *Journal of Bone and Joint Surgery,* **58A,** 796–800.

Lehmman W., Menche D., Grant A., Normal A. & Pugh J. (1984) The problem of evaluating *in situ* pinning of SCFE: An experimental model and review of 63 cases. *Journal of Paediatric Orthopaedics,* **4,** 297–303.

Litchman H. & Duffy J. (1984) Slipped capital femoral epiphysis: Factors affecting shear forces on the epiphyseal plate. *Journal of Paediatric Orthopaedics,* **4**, 745–8.

Morrissey R., Steele R. & Gerdes M. (1983) Localized immune complexes and slipped upper femoral epiphysis. *Journal of Bone and Joint Surgery,* **65B**, 574–9.

Ninomiya S., Nagasaka Y. & Tagawa H. (1976) Slipped capital femoral epiphysis: A study of 68 cases in the Eastern Half Area of Japan. *Clinical Orthopaedics and Related Research,* **119**, 172–6.

O'Brien E. & Fahey J. (1977) Remodelling of the femoral neck after *in situ* pinning for slipped capital epiphysis. *Journal of Bone and Joint Surgery,* **59A**, 62–8.

Orofino G., Innis J. & Lowry C. (1960) Slipped capital femoral epiphysis in Negroes. *Journal of Bone and Joint Surgery,* **42A**, 1023–79.

Poland J. (1898) *Traumatic Separation of the Epiphysis.* Smith, Elder & Co., London.

Puri R., Smith C. S., Malhotra D., Williams A., Owen R. & Harris F. (1985) Slipped upper femoral epiphysis and primary juvenile hypothyroidism. *Journal of Bone and Joint Surgery,* **67B**, 14–20.

Rao J., Francis A. & Siwek C. (1984) The treatment of chronic slipped capital femoral epiphysis by biplane osteotomy. *Journal of Bone and Joint Surgery,* **66A**, 1169–75.

Ratliffe A. (1968) Traumatic separation of the upper femoral epiphysis in young children. *Journal of Bone and Joint Surgery,* **50B**, 757–70.

Rennie A. (1982) The inheritance of slipped upper femoral epiphysis. *Journal of Bone and Joint Surgery,* **64B**, 180–4.

Salvati E., Robinson H. & O'Dowd T. (1980) Southwicks osteotomy for severe SCFE: Results and complications. *Journal of Bone and Joint Surgery,* **62A**, 561–9.

Southwick W. O. (1967) Osteotomy through the lesser trochanter for slipped capital femoral epiphysis. *Journal of Bone and Joint Surgery,* **49A**, 807–34.

Southwick W. O. (1984) Slipped capital femoral epiphysis (Editorial). *Journal of Bone and Joint Surgery,* **66A**, 1151.

Weiner D., Weiner S., Melby A. & Hoyt W. (1984) A 30- year experience with bone graft epiphysiodesis in the treatment of SCFE. *Journal of Paediatric Orthopaedics,* **4**, 145–52.

Wiberg G. (1959) Considerations on the surgical treatment of slipped epiphysis with special reference to nail fixation. *Journal of Bone and Joint Surgery,* **91A**, 253–61.

Wilson P., Jacobs B. & Schecter L. (1965) Slipped capital femoral epiphysis: An end result study. *Journal of Bone and Joint Surgery,* **47A**, 1128–45.

Wright W. & King D. (1956) The treatment of slipped capital femoral epiphysis. *American Journal of Surgery,* **91**, 894–9.

9

Fractures Around the Hip

N. J. BLOCKEY

Fractures around the hip in children comprise perhaps 1–2% of the total hip fractures with which a surgeon is expected to deal. The femoral neck in normal infants and children is strong so that major violence is necessary to fracture the bone in this region. Whilst avascular necrosis and nonunion are prominent problems, as they are in the adult, coxa vara and other effects of distorted femoral growth must be added to the list of complications in children. From a practical point of view, the aim of treatment is to reduce the fracture and to hold it reduced such that union will occur within 12–16 weeks. This must be accomplished without damage to the precarious blood supply of the femoral head and with minimal interference to the epiphyseal growth plate.

As in all difficult fractures in children, the complication rate seems higher where operative treatment has been undertaken or multiple manipulations performed. Judgment is required to determine whether the position achieved after a competent manipulation is acceptable or whether open reduction, with its additional complications, should be performed. Another potential cause of disaster is to attempt to manage such fractures with adult size instruments and devices, for example the use of a Smith–Peterson nail in a child's femoral neck; this leads to the conclusion that these fracutres should only be managed in a children's hospital or in a unit familiar with the care of young patients and by surgeons with a knowledge of longterm effects of growth and remodelling. Finally, operations designed to remedy the longterm effects of these fractures which simply seem a good idea, but whose prognosis is not known are best avoided.

Classification

Delbet's (1929) simple classification with the approximate percentage incidence is as follows:

Type I   Transepiphyseal, with or without dislocation of the femoral head (3%)
Type II   Transcervical (50%)
Type III Cervico-intertrochanteric (37%)
Type IV   Intertrochanteric (10%)

Review of literature

The three papers analysing the problems encountered worldwide in these injuries and worthy of close study emanate from the United Kingdom, the United States and Hong Kong. Ratliff (1962) published his deliberations on 73 cases of femoral neck fractures in children under the age of 17 years. Forty-three surgeons contributed cases to the study and he added 19 which he had personally treated. The classifications and the incidence of the various types of fracture was similar to that stated above. Avascular necrosis was the commonest serious complication occuring in 42%. It was most common in displaced transcervical fractures and was always evident radiologically within one year. In half the affected cases there was collapse of the whole proximal fragment, the others having either necrosis of only the neck fragment, leaving the epiphysis uninvolved, or patchy necrosis of the superior segment of the epiphysis (Fig. 9.1). The prognosis in the former group was uniformly poor regardless of the method of treatment of the original fracture. In a later publication (Ratliff 1970) the same author enlarged his experience to 132 cases. The overall proportion of the various types of fractures was the same as in the original series. Seventy-one per cent developed complications, 38% nonunion, 15% developed coxa vara and an alarming 20% developed premature epiphyseal fusion. This included six children who, due to prolonged immobilization, developed premature fusion at the lower end of the femur. From this detailed analysis and follow-up he drew tentative conclusions as to how best to manage these injuries. For undisplaced fractures a plaster hip spica was recommended. Displaced transcervical fractures had given such disappointing results in the patients he had studied that for them he suggested subtrochanteric osteotomy. When this was performed as a primary procedure it gave two good and two poor results in four patients and, when used because primary treatment had failed, the operation gave eight reasonably good final results out of ten hips he described as 'otherwise hopeless'. His dissatisfaction with the reduction and fixation of displaced

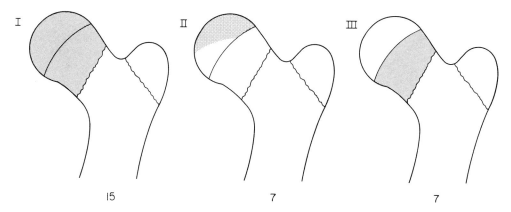

I   II   III

15   7   7

Fig. 9.1 Types of avascular necrosis seen in the 29 cases among 73 children's femoral neck fractures (modified from Ratliff 1962).

transcervical fractures arose, it would appear, because fixation was attempted using inappropriate devices (*see* second paragraph) leading to the conclusion that, as in the adult femoral neck, the bad results of fixation are the results of bad fixation.

Canale and Bourland (1977) described another large series of children's femoral neck fractures and followed 61 such fractures in 60 children into adult life. The average age at the time of fracture in this Campbell clinic series was 9.7 years and the follow-up was from 3 to 53 years (average 17.0 years) when 55% had good results 20% fair and 25% poor. In Type I fractures their recommendation was to try manipulation only. If this fails proceed to open reduction. In either case fixation with Knowles pins is advised. Four out of five of their Type I fracture dislocations required open reduction and all five developed avascular necrosis resulting in degenerative arthritis in adult life in four. For Type II and III fractures their recommendation is gentle closed manipulation and the insertion of Knowles pins. Although 14 of the 22 displaced fractures in their groups developed avasuclar necrosis it is unlikely that the insertion of pins worsened the outlook because, of four treated by manipulation and plaster spica fixation, three developed avasuclar necrosis. In adult life these fourteen gave seven poor and six fair results.

Lam (1971) described his experience in Hong Kong where he had treated and followed up 37 transcervical fractures. Twenty were displaced. Although he considered that the problem of these fractures was still unsolved, he felt that, whereas in younger children closed manipulation and spica fixation gave satisfactory results, in older age groups internal fixation was necessary. In Lam's hands this policy resulted in 17% developing avascular necrosis and this is more in accord with the current Glasgow teaching.

Canale and King (1984) made the point that, whilst the rate of avascular necrosis was the same in their series as in Lam's, the higher incidence of union and the smaller proportion developing coxa vara suggested that fixation with the correct appliance is both desirable and effective. For this reason they advocate internal fixation, usually with Knowles pins, for both displaced and undisplaced transcervical fractures.

This review of previous work plus some personal experience leads to the following practical guidance.

Principles of treatment

Avascular necrosis is probably due to initial displacement and can not be avoided by treatment. That said, however, this complication can also be caused by surgical exposure of the fractured femoral neck. In an imperfectly reduced fracture, a decision must be made whether to open the neck and achieve anatomical reduction, thereby increasing the possibility of avascular necrosis, or to accept the imperfect position increasing the likelihood of delayed union or late development of coxa vara. Delayed and nonunion and the dreaded distal femoral epiphyseal arrest can be avoided by internal fixation and the avoidance of over long immobilization. If things go wrong subtrochanteric displacement osteotomy without internal fixation has been shown to give satisfactory results provided that the upper end of the femoral shaft is placed and held beneath the fracture site. These points are illustrated in the following examples: Fig. 9.2 shows an anteroposterior radiograph of the hip of a child aged two presenting two weeks after a severe fall. This delay made an attempt at anatomical reduction dangerous. A displacement osteotomy was performed and after three months in a one-and-a-half hip spica, union occurred without avascular necrosis. Fig. 9.3 shows Type I transepiphyseal separation ending

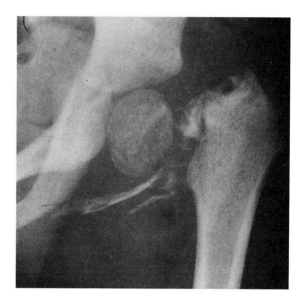

Fig. 9.2 A transcervical fracture in a child of 2 years.

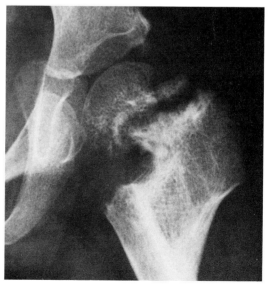

Fig. 9.3 An example of a type I transepiphyseal separation.

up with slight shortening. Fig. 9.4a is a postreduction radiograph of the hip of a child aged four with a displaced transcervical fracture. While imperfect, it was decided for the reasons given to immobilize the hip in this position for eight weeks. Fig. 9.4b is the picture then revealed showing avascular necrosis of the proximal neck fragment and slight recurrence of displacement without any sign of union. This was felt to be unacceptable. The fracture was opened, soft tissue was removed from the fracture site, the fracture was reduced and held reduced by two threaded

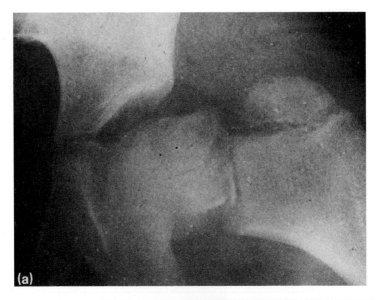

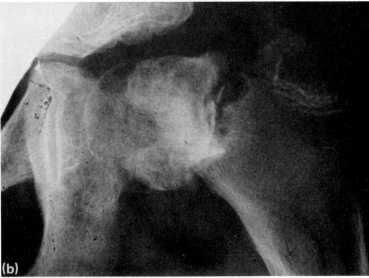

Fig. 9.4 (a) Postreduction radiograph of hip in child (aged 4 years) with displaced transcervical fracture. (b) Avascular necrosis of proximal neck fragment.

Moore's pins (Fig. 9.4c). This led to union in a further eight weeks with residual coxa vara (Fig. 9.4d). Fig. 9.5a shows a basal comminuted fracture. Traction, abduction and slight internal rotation produced an acceptable position (Fig. 9.5b). This was not opened or fixed because, over the following 8 weeks, serial radiographs showed no change in position. After 12 weeks the fracture united without complications (Fig. 9.5c). Study of the radiographs of Figs. 9.4a and 9.5b show the author's opinion of what is acceptable manipulative reduction and what is not.

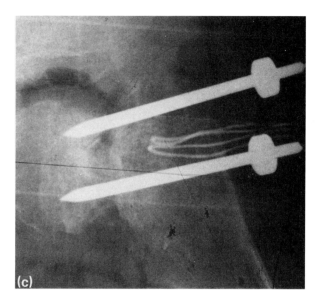

Fig. 9.4 (c) After removal of soft tissue the fracture was reduced and held by two threaded Moore's pins.

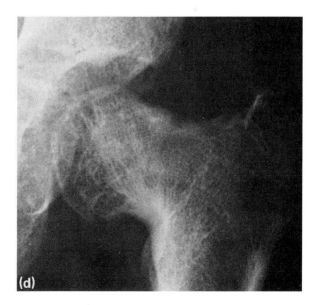

Fig. 9.4 (d) Eight weeks later there is union with residual coxa vara.

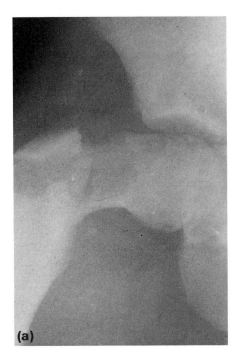

Fig. 9.5 (a) A basal comminuted fracture.

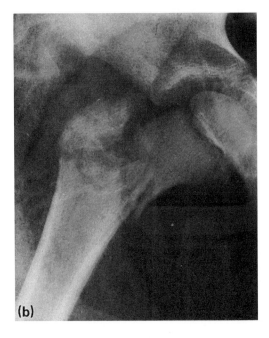

(b) Postreduction.

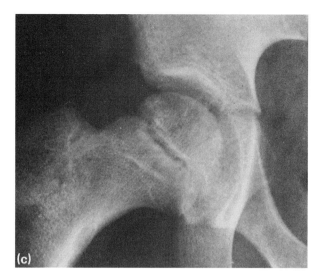

(c) Union at 12 weeks.

Guidelines

Care for the patient in a children's unit and do not tackle the problem without skilled anaesthesia, image intensification, a Hawley table and instruments and appliances geared to children's bones.

Attempt a manipulation on the Hawley table remembering that, as for the adult, abduction and slight internal rotation is most often necessary for reduction. Ignore the greater trochanter. Get the neck shaft angle correct and, if satifactory, hold the leg in full abduction and insert two pins. Use small diameter 5/64 inch or 2 mm Steinmann pins or an introducer or a threaded cannulated screw. Kirschner wires are too thin and 4 mm Steinmann pins too thick. Threaded Knowles pins of 3.2 mm shaft diameter are often suitable in a bigger child. Smith–Peterson pins, Pugh or Jewett nails or indeed any device that requires hammering into the epiphysis foretell disaster. For basal fractures use the Coventry infant lag screw instruments by Howmedica. Do not subsequently immobilize in plaster for longer than four months.

If manipulative reduction is impossible open the fracture through a Watson-Jones approach, remove interposed soft tissue and retrograde the pins out through the trochanter. Then, under direct vision, close the fracture and push the pins right into the head. If things go wrong perform a subtrochanteric osteotomy.

It should be possible by these methods to avoid all complications except avasular necrosis. If this occurs accept it, wait for union and mobilize nonweightbearing for a year. If total avascular necrosis of the proximal segment ensues, do not attempt to revascularize it by grafts. This never works, the acetabulum becomes distorted secondary to the femoral head collapse and the hip is doomed.

If coxa vara with a final neck shaft angle less than 100° is seen after union, perform a valgus osteotomy by excising a laterally based wedge, i.e. a closing wedge, and rigidly fix with a Coventry screw and plate. Osteotomies opening medially are impossible.

Summary

These fractures result from major trauma. In infants child abuse is sometimes responsible. Look out of other injuries. Use precise techniques as far as possible and the instruments mentioned. All types of III and IV fractures should do well with rigid internal fixation using a cannulated screw and lateral plate. Do not aim too high. It is far better to get union with some coxa vara than total avascular necrosis due to too forcible retraction.

References

Canale S. T. & King R. E. (1984) In *Fractures in Children* (Rockwood C. A., Wilkins K. E. and King R. E. eds.). J. B. Lippincott Company, Philadelphia.

Canale S. T. & Bourland W. L. (1977) Fracture of the neck and intertrochanteric region of the femur in children. *Journal of Bone and Joint Surgery,* **59A,** 431–43.

Delbet P. quoted in Colonna P. (1929) *American Journal of Surgery,* **6,** 793.

Lam S. F. (1971) Fractures of the neck of the femur in children. *Journal of Bone and Joint Surgery,* **53A,** 1165–79.

Ratliff A. H. C. (1962) Fractures of the neck of the femur in children. *Journal of Bone and Joint Surgery,* **44B,** 528–42.

Ratliff A. H. C. (1970) Complications after fractures of the femoral neck in children and their treatment. *Journal of Bone and Joint Surgery,* **55B,** 175.

10

The Hip in Neuromuscular Disorders

G. C. BENNET & G. A. EVANS

Myelomeningocele

Prior to the introduction of an effective means of controlling hydrocephalus, only 10–15% of children with myelomeningocele survived beyond childhood, these invariably being the less severely affected cases (Asher & Olson 1983). The availability of CSF shunting, combined with the use of antibiotics, has now made survival the rule rather than the exception. Once survival was assured, treatment of deformities in these children became possible. Based on experience gained in the management of poliomyelitis and traumatic paraplegia, all were aggressively treated with a combination of surgery and bracing in the expectation that they would become, and remain, ambulant (Lorber 1971). These hopes did not materialize. It slowly became apparent that, because of their multiple handicaps, they did less well than had originally been anticipated. A more realistic approach gradually emerged. The yardstick of success became the effectiveness of a treatment in improving the child's quality of life, rather than the technical success of the procedure or merely prolonged survival. Selection began to be practised, not only from an orthopaedic point of view, but in the overall management of the condition. At birth those children with features which bode ill for their future quality of life did not receive active treatment, whereas those in whom no such adverse factors were present were treated aggressively with closure of the back and CSF shunting. Screening for the disorder is now standard antenatal care. All pregnant women have their serum alphafetoprotein levels measured between the sixteenth and eighteenth weeks of pregnancy. This, combined with the use of ultrasound and amniocentesis when raised values are found, allows termination to be offered to those with an affected fetus. By such means the number of cases of spina bifida cystica arising in a population can be dramatically reduced.

The realism that has been applied to the care of these children is equally applicable to their orthopaedic management in general and to their hip problems in particular. Whilst the principles governing the basic approach to such problems have gained some degree of acceptance, the methods by which the agreed goals are obtained are far less clearly defined. Before discussing these, however, the other more general problems associated with myelomeningocele will be briefly reviewed so as to put the hip problems into their proper perspective.

Although, if present, hydrocephalus can normally be kept under control by shunting procedures, such control is not always complete. Repeated changes of malfunctioning drainage systems may adversely affect the patient's cerebral function. Abnormalities of the spinal cord proximal to the back lesion can result in less than perfect function in the upper limbs and may affect the child's ability to use walking aids. Incontinence of bladder and bowel is almost invariably present and, unless this is properly controlled, social integration will be impossible. Spinal deformity, obesity, and lack of sensation, all combine to make the orthopaedic treatment of these unfortunate children far from straightforward. Even the abnormalities in the spinal cord are subject to variation. Thus, whilst the lesion may produce a picture akin to that of adult paraplegia in the lower limbs, the presence of foot deformities in an otherwise paralysed limb may signal the existence of an area of reflex activity distal to the level of paralysis (Stark & Baker 1967). The same authors also describe cases in which descending tracts pass through the spinal lesion to produce an intact area of supply to part of the limb distal to the paralysed segment. To further complicate matters, the two limbs may be affected asymmetrically. Although a true hemimyelomeningocele producing paralysis in one limb is rare, minor variations of activity between the two sides, particularly below the knee, are not uncommon (Huff & Ramsay 1978).

The genesis of deformity

Deformity develops at the hip because of imbalance between muscle groups acting across the joint. If for example, the muscles on one side are active, whether under voluntary control or not, and the antagonists are either not active or not acting as strongly, then deformity will result. The unopposed activity of a muscle eventually results in its shortening whilst, on the other hand, constant stretching produces lengthening of its antagonist which causes it to be put at an increasing mechanical disadvantage. This means that once the process of deformation has started it becomes self perpetuating. Deformity will not result if all muscles are either nomally active or if none are active and the limb is flail.

The pattern of muscular activity in the lower limbs in myelomeningocele is dictated by the level of the spinal lesion, i.e. the neurosegmental level. Thus, in a thoracic lesion, that is at the level of T12 or above, the legs are completely flail. An L1/2 lesion is characterized by good hip flexion power and weak adduction whereas, at L3/4, in addition to normal function in the hip flexors and adductors, activity will be present in the quadriceps and medial hamstrings. Not until the L5 level is reached does hip abduction become possible and only in a sacral lesion is hip extension present. The pattern of muscular activity dictates the deformities that will develop. Thus unopposed hip flexion causes the limb to lie in flexion, abduction and external rotation whilst the addition of adductor activity produces flexion and adduction leading to subluxation and dislocation. Only once power develops in the hip abductors, that is at L5, does the risk of this happening diminish.

Bony deformity develops secondary to deformity in the soft tissues. Paralysis of hip abduction leads to diminished growth on the lateral side of the femoral neck resulting in coxa valga. Other abnormalities commonly found in the proximal femur are osteoporosis and elongation ·of the neck — both being the result of reduced mechanical stress across the joint (Fig. 10.1). Unless the hip is dislocated at birth acetabular development is normally good and, unlike congenital dislocation of the hip, dysplasia develops only after longstanding dislocation. This of course suggests that its development can be prevented by early active treatment.

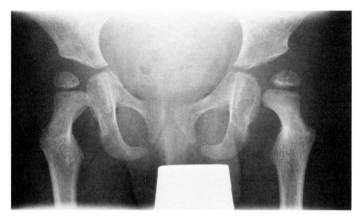

Fig. 10.1 An anteroposterior radiograph of the hips in myelomeningocele. The femoral necks are thin, elongated and in a valgus position.

Prediction of function

The treatment of any disorder must be based upon a knowledge of its natural history and that of any deformity in the knowledge of what the effect of the deformity would be upon the child's ultimate capabilities if it were left untreated. Only then can the potentially beneficial effects of treatment be assessed. In most cases justification for the treatment of hip deformities lies in the effect such deformities have upon mobility. This in turn is dependent upon many factors some of which can be influenced by treatment and some of which cannot. Before considering these, however, it should be first be borne in mind that walking is not an end in itself. It must be useful and offer some benefits over the function that can be attained in a wheelchair. Only then will it be maintained. All children with spina bifida will, given appropriate bracing, walk and indeed should be encouraged to do so. Not all will continue walking in adult life. There is obviously no point in launching into a series of ever more complicated surgical procedures in a child who, at the end of the day, will lead a wheelchair existance. They will have been exposed to all the risks of major surgery and its attendant disruption of normal schooling, independence training and family life for no perceptible potential gain. Far better to have anticipated their adult capabilities, and therefore their needs, and tailored their treatment towards that goal. Obviously the earlier an assessment of their ultimate function can be made the more effective and least disruptive can the treatment be. Fortunately certain guidelines can be used for this purpose, the most important of these being the neurosegmental level. All other factors are of secondary importance. The more muscles that are functional the more likely it is that the child will walk and will continue to do so. Thus, with higher neurosegmental levels, the chances of continued ambulation are lower than in those with more distal lesions. This, however, is not an absolute criterion for, even within apparently similar neurosegmental levels, there may be some variation in the motor power of functioning muscles (Menelaus 1980). The majority of children who continue to walk have lesions at or below L3, that is they have functioning quadriceps (Table 10.1). Even then, only those children who become community walkers during childhood will maintain their walking ability in adult life. Therapeutic or household walking tends to be a transitory phase and at maturity such children normally opt for a wheelchair existence (Fiewell *et al.* 1978).

Table 10.1 Percentage of community walkers according to the neurosegmental level
(after Stillwell & Menelaus 1983)

Neurosegmental level	Stillwell & Menelaus	Desouza & Carroll	Fiewell et al.	Hoffer et al.
Thoracic (%)	33	0	0	0
High lumbar	30	10	26	31
Low lumbar	95	30	76	38
Sacral	100	53	82	100
Age range in years	15–31	12–26	6–29	5–42
Number of cases	80	68	76	56

Although factors other than the neurosegmental level are of much less importance, they at least can be modified by treatment. Only if the neurosegmental level is compatible with continued walking however, can permanent improvement as a result of their alteration be anticipated.

Whether or not the femoral head is correctly positioned in the acetabulum seems to make little difference either to walking ability or the orthotic requirements of a child (Fiewell *et al.* 1978, Stillwell & Menelaus 1983, Erken 1984). Nor does it correlate with the range of movement of the joint (Fiewell *et al.* 1978). Hip deformity on the other hand does seem to have an adverse affect on walking ability. Asher and Olsen (1983) found fixed flexion deformities to be the only significant variable in the walking capabilities of those with an L3/4 neurosegmental level. Stillwell & Menelaus (1983) reported similar findings. Other less important factors, often not evident until later childhood, include obesity, scoliosis, pelvic obliquity and the character of the child, this last accounting for both under and over achievement.

With these in mind realistic goals can be set for each child and this in turn allows realistic treatment, set within the confines of these goals, to be offered to suit their individual needs. (Menelaus 1976). In practical terms this means that only those children with good walking potential should be subjected to radical hip surgery, whereas limited muscle releases are indicated in the more severely affected child. If the decision to operate is made, the subsequent surgical planning should be in line with the condensed management described by (Menelaus 1980). All necessary procedures on the lower limbs should be performed at one session, so as to allow for the minimal possible period of postoperative immobilization and least disruption to the child's life.

Assessment

If these facts are kept in mind, assessment of the child becomes much simpler. Obviously there are difficulties in the first year of life. During this time the mere presence of movement does not mean that a muscle is under voluntary control. By repeated testing and observation of the baby's posture (as well as listening to the parents) a fairly accurate record of motor activity can be obtained by the age of one and certainly by the age of two, an accurate prediction of the child's ultimate function can be made. As soon as the muscle pattern has been established then surgery, if indicated, can be undertaken with safety. Such early surgery can be limited to the soft tissues as secondary bony deformities have not usually developed and indeed successful surgery at this age should prevent their doing so.

The aims of assessment can be categorized under three headings:

1   What is its general health of the child? Is there a valve *in situ* and is it giving any trouble? Are there any infections present, particularly in the urinary tract? Are there any skin sores? What is the renal function? How are the child and parents coping? What schooling arrangements are anticipated, etc.
2   What is the neurosegmental level? Assess this from both a motor and sensory point of view, although the latter is possible only in the older child.
3   Assess and record the child's deformities. This should be done not only at the hip but in the rest of the lower limbs, the spine and pelvis.

The information obtained by such an assessment should allow an appreciation of the child's present general physical status to be made, its likely future walking capabilities and, if deformities are indeed present around the hip, how aggressively they should be treated.

Hip deformities

These include: coxa vara
                fixed flexion deformity
                flexion/abduction/external rotation
                  deformity
                subluxation/dislocation

Coxa vara

This deformity may arise in one of three ways (Weisl 1983):

1 Separation of the upper femoral epiphysis (Fig. 10.2).

This probably occurs due to a combination of an abnormal physeal plate and trauma. There is seldom a history of significant trauma and it seems more likely that relatively minor trauma, perhaps sustained while stretching an abduction contracture (Dias 1983), is the cause. Nonunion is the rule.

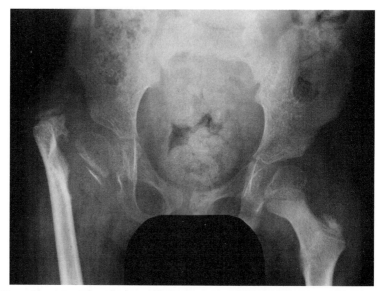

Fig. 10.2 Upper femoral epiphysiolysis producing coxa vara. This was an incidental finding and did not appear to have an adverse effect on the child's gait. There was no history of trauma.

2 Fracture of the femoral neck (Fig. 10.3).

This is a not uncommon occurrence, particularly after a period of immobilization in a hip spica. If it is extracapsular then healing with excessive callus, as is characteristically found in paraplegia, is likely. Avascular necrosis is rare, presumably reflecting the minor degree of trauma required to produce such fractures.

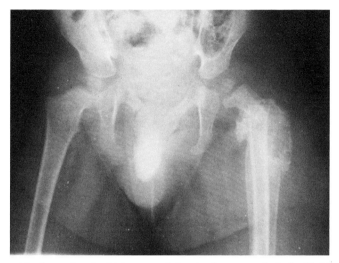

Fig. 10.3 Fracture of the femoral neck which occurred shortly after removal of a double hip spica. Note the excessive callus typically found in myelomeningocele.

3 Avascular necrosis (Fig. 10.4).

This can be produced by excessive abduction, whether in a hip spica or broomstick type plaster, in the presence of adductor tightness (Carroll & Sharrard 1972). The changes may prove to be transient or may result in the later development of coxa vara.

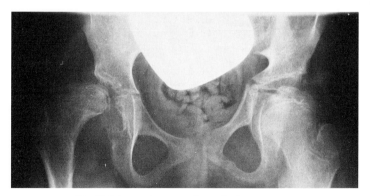

Fig. 10.4 Avascular necrosis producing coxa vara.

In spite of their occasionally alarming radiographic appearance, none of these lesions requires surgical intervention for the simple reason that they do not appear to increase the child's handicap nor do they cause any deterioration in their mobility.

Fixed flexion deformity (Fig. 10.5)

Fixed flexion deformity at the hip can be found in almost any child with a myelomeningocele whatever the neurosegmental level. Indeed it may even occur in children with completely flail hips as a result of prolonged sitting in a wheelchair. Although usually assessed clinically by the Thomas test, this may be difficult, if not impossible to perform in the presence of fixed deformities, particularly a kyphosis, in the lumbar spine. A more effective method is shown in Fig. 10.6. In those children who adopt a wheelchair existance, the presence of a fixed flexion deformity, whilst inevitable, is not necessarily detrimental to their function. Correction is not indicated as it will recur. In those that remain mobile, however, it does impair walking ability and, as we have already seen, is strongly correlated

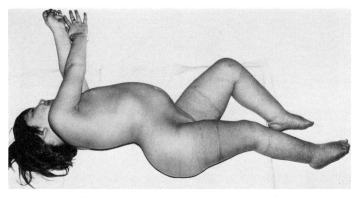

Fig. 10.5 Severe bilateral fixed flexion deformities. Note the poor distal peripheral circulation typically found in spina bifida.

with nonambulation (Stillwell & Menelaus 1983). In the newborn child fixed flexion of 20–30° is normal. This gradually decreases over the first few months of life but, in the presence of muscle imbalance, however, this resolution does not take place. In such cases the use of a total body splint to hold the hips in extension has been advocated (Schaffer & Dias 1983). We have not had much success with this approach and now prefer to undertake surgical correction if the deformity cannot be controlled with physiotherapy. The procedure may be undertaken at any age, but the chances of success become less with increasing age. Correction is achieved by an anterior hip release, sometimes combined with release of the adductors.

Through a transverse groin incision 2 cm distal to the adductor tubercle, the lesser trochanter is exposed and 1 cm of the psoas tendon excised. This wound is packed with a swab whilst a second Smith–Peterson incision is made. The iliac apophysis is split and the tight muscles are allowed to retract down the sides of the iliac bone. Any remaining tight anterior structures are then released as necessary, safeguarding only the neurovascular bundle. Whilst the aim is to obtain full extension, this is often not achieved, but nevertheless significant reduction can be obtained. Postoperatively the child is placed in a double hip spica with the hips

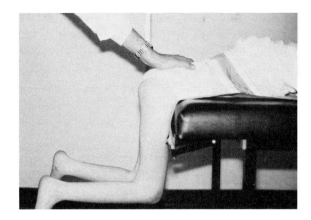

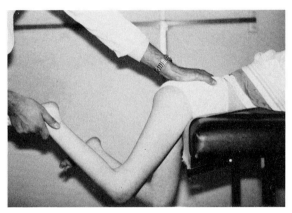

Fig. 10.6 Testing for fixed flexion deformity. The child is positioned prone with the legs hanging over the edge of the examination couch (top). With one hand on the pelvis one hip is extended. The angle the thigh makes with the horizontal when the pelvis begins to rotate, is the degree of fixed flexion.

in extension for six weeks, with an hour or two weightbearing each day.

Whilst it is said that up to 50° fixed flexion can be corrected by such means, it is obviously more effective when done earlier for less severe deformities (Menelaus 1980). In more severe deformities an extension osteotomy is necessary. We have not used this procedure as, by the time the deformity has become so severe, the potential functional gain has never appeared sufficient to risk the possible adverse effect such a procedure might have on sitting.

Flexion/abduction and external rotation deformity (Fig. 10.7)

This pattern of deformity arises in upper lumbar lesions when only the hip flexors are working. The muscle action has much the same effect as putting a child in a Pavlik harness with hip flexion producing passive abduction and external rotation. If the position becomes fixed then fitting of the appropriate orthoses becomes impossible. As these children require hip/knee/ankle/foot orthoses, even slight abduction contractures will lead, in the active child, to repeated breaking of the hip joint of the orthosis. Whilst it is acknowledged that few of these children maintain ambulation in adult life, it is nevertheless worthwhile correcting the deformity early on if parental manipulations fail to do so as not to would deprive them of their childhood mobility. Early treatment consists of wrapping a pinned pillowcase around the child's legs whilst it is resting and at night so as to keep them extended. If this does not prove to be effective, then surgical correction must be considered. The adoption of a flexed externally rotated position moulds away the normal anteversion of the femoral neck and indeed retroversion may be present

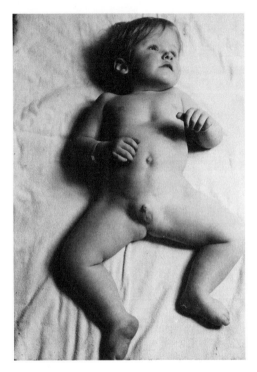

Fig. 10.7 Flexion/abduction/ external rotation contracture in a boy with lower limb activity only in the hip flexors.

(Menelaus 1980). Schaffer and Dias (1983) demonstrated this in two such hips documented by CT scan. Because of its presence the authors would concur with Menelaus (1980) that it is illogical to attempt to correct the deformity by derotation osteotomy and rather that it should be done by a soft tissue release. Such a release consists of division of the active hip flexors, as previously described, and in addition, if necessary, the tight abductors by releasing the tensor fascia lata at its origin as well as any other tight lateral structures found at operation, until complete correction is obtained. External rotation can be corrected by division of the tight short external rotators and hip capsule posteriorly, combined with anterior capsular reefing (Menelaus 1980).

Subluxation/dislocation

According to Sharrard (1971) more than half the children with myelomeningocele will develop subluxation or dislocation of the hip. This estimate is in agreement with the figures of Ramsay (1978), who, in a study of 130 myelomeningocele hips, found 73 to be unstable, 48 being subluxed and 25 dislocated.

The incidence of instability is in direct proportion to the degree of muscle imbalance. Thus it is less common in an L1/2 lesion where the adductors are acting only weakly than at the L3/4 level where there is normal adductor power, but still none in the abductors.

The importance of hip subluxation or dislocation lies not in its mere presence, but in its effect on the child's walking or sitting ability. As has already been stated, there appears to be no correlation between the position of the hip, that is, whether it is reduced or not, and its range of motion (Carroll & Sharrard 1972). Nor indeed does subluxation or dislocation appear to adversely affect walking ability, particularly in children who wear long leg calipers. In view of this, there can be no doubt that a dislocated mobile hip is a preferable situation to a reduced stiff one. That said, however, a unilateral dislocation undoubtedly does result in a leg length discrepancy, poor sitting balance and perhaps, pelvic obliquity and scoliosis (Fig. 10.8).

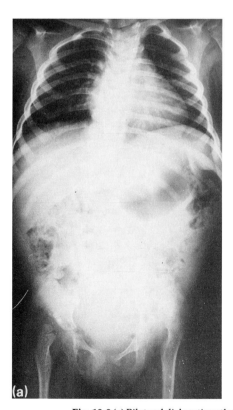
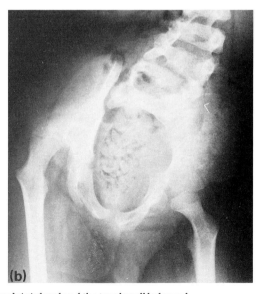

Fig. 10.8 (a) Bilateral dislocation: the pelvis is level and the trunk well balanced.
(b) Unilateral dislocation: there is marked pelvic obliquity. The effect this will have in both sitting and walking is evident.

Treatment is governed by the assessment of the child's ultimate potential. It may be aimed at reducing the hip, correcting the bony abnormalities and restoring muscle imbalance or alternatively merely eliminating deformity by simple soft tissue releases. In either case, useful function, even if it is only passive motion, should never be put at risk. The most difficult aspect in the management of hip stability in spina bifida lies in matching the correct procedure to a particular child. Obviously, the more the potential benefit, the more extensive the surgery may be, always mindful that the achievement of a stable posture rather than a good radiographic appearance is the aim. The first prerequisite in selection is a knowledge of the longterm walking potential of the child. In this an accurate assessment of the neurosegmental level is vital. As we have already discussed, this is difficult before the age of one so that it is better to postpone surgery until after then in the anticipation of achieving more predictable results. On the other hand, beyond the age of three, bony surgery to treat secondary abnormalities may well be required (Drennan 1983), and beyond the age of five, the results of surgical intervention become less good and improvement in function less likely (Jackson *et al.* 1979). The ideal age for surgery then is when they are old enough to assess properly, but before the development of secondary bony changes, usually between the ages of eighteen months and three years.

In practical terms what does this mean? Bilaterally dislocated or subluxed hips in children with upper lumbar lesions who are unlikely to continue independent walking are best left and reduction not attempted. In them simple soft tissue releases to rid them of deformity is all that is required. On the other hand a unilateral dislocation in a child with a low lumbar neurosegmental level, and thus with good walking potential, should, in the absence of contraindications, be treated aggressively with whatever procedures are required to attain and maintain reduction. These are the simple decisions. Less clear-cut is the management of unilateral dislocation in the upper lumbar child and the bilateral dislocation in a child with good walking potential. We are of the opinion that, even in a child who is likely to adopt a wheelchair existence, a unilateral dislocation is best reduced. Whilst leg length discrepancy in them is of little importance, the adverse effect of the dislocation on sitting posture probably justifies treatment. In bilateral dislocations in a potentially independent child, the decision is difficult. Because of the high incidence of attendant complications and the risk of producing asymmetry due to failure of reduction on one side, we would not advise attempted reduction. In each case the individual circumstances of the child must be considered. Severe spinal deformity, acetabular dysplasia, as is found in a congenitally dislocated hip, spasticity or mental retardation might all militate against a successful result and alter the decision in a particular case.

Closed treatment

Closed methods of treatment are not now widely used or advocated perhaps because they do not seem to work. Dias (1983) cites 40 hips treated by closed manipulation followed by a period of immobilization in a hip spica. With one exception all progressively subluxed and were dislocated at follow-up. Prophylactic splinting in the first year of life, however, still receives some support. The rationale behind its continued use is to try to prevent deformity occurring whilst waiting until the child is old enough for a decision to be made with regard to operative treatment. The splint described by McKibben (1973) is based on the Bachelor position of abduction and internal rotation. By this means the psoas, the principle deforming force, is kept on stretch. Drennan (1973) and Dias (1983) have also advocated the use of early splintage both of them favouring an abduction type body orthosis.

There are drawbacks, however, to their use. In the neonate, treatment of hip instability is obviously of a low priority, taking second place to the management of the spinal lesion and developing hydrocephalus. Later, complications may arise. Skin sores, fractures and fixed deformities are all potential pitfalls. The effect of the use of such splintage on parents should not be underestimated. They are already overwhelmed by their tragedy and the use of a splint may add yet one more burden at a particularly difficult time. All this, however, might be set aside if the use of splintage were shown to be effective. Reduction of a neurological dislocation of the hip is not usually difficult, although maintaining the reduction is. The claim that their use simplifies subsequent operation, should it be necessary, is not a strong one. Similarly, unless muscle imbalance is corrected, which it cannot be by closed methods, maintenance of reduction is unlikely. What results are available would seem to support this view. For these reasons we would not advocate their use.

Soft tissue procedures

The aim of any soft tissue procedure is to restore muscle balance. This may be achieved either by weakening a stronger muscle by a simple release, or reinforcing a weaker one by the transfer of a more active muscle. (Obviously this removes the deforming effect of the transferred muscle in the process.)

Soft tissue release

Simple division of the deforming muscles, namely the adductors and iliopsoas, has usually been reserved for patients with upper lumbar lesions. In them, because of variable activity in the adductors, the imbalance is not usually as severe as when the adductors are normally active. Additionally, the likelihood of their continuing to have independent mobility is low. The procedure consists of release of the psoas tendon and part of the adductors through a medial groin incision. Through a transverse incision some 2 cm below the adductor tubercle, the fascia is split longitudinally to expose first the tendon of adductor longus. Using finger dissection, this is delivered into the wound and divided using diathermy. By the same method the gracilis, a surprisingly large muscle is delivered and similarly treated. Once again using a finger, the lesser trochanter is palpated by passing the finger immediately anterior to the adductor brevis. A McDonald dissector passed anterior to the shaft of the femur at the level of the lesser trochanter and retracted laterally exposes the lesser trochanter and attached psoas tendon. The tendon is freed of soft tissue by blunt dissection and a 1 cm section excised. A good range of abduction should then be possible. If some restriction remains, further sectioning of the adductors is indicated until the desired correction has been achieved.

The results of this method have previously been reported as unreliable although only in small numbers. Dias (1978) found that redislocation occurred in 7 out of 8 hips treated by medial release and Sharrard (1964) described redislocation occurring in five out of six similarly treated at birth. The authors' results have certainly been rather better. The procedure has been performed on 23 hips in 19 patients with the average age at operation being three years. The follow-up ranged from two to eleven years with an average of 7.6 years. The outcome is shown in Table 10.2. Postoperatively only 2 patients had significant fixed flexion deformities, both of these being secondary to bony ankylosis.

Table 10.2 The results of soft tissue release in hip instability.

Upper lumbar	*11 patients*	*14 tenotomies*
Pre-op.	7 dislocated	7 unstable
Post-op.	4 reduced	6 reduced
Lower lumbar	*7 patients*	*9 tenotomies*
Pre-op.	6 dislocated	3 unstable
Post-op.		All but 1 reduced

Muscle transfers

Mustard iliopsoas transfer

In this procedure (Mustard 1959) the tendon of the iliopsoas is transferred laterally, from the lesser to the greater trochanter, thus changing its action from being predominantly one of flexion to one of abduction although, as it still crosses anterior to the hip joint, it retains some of its flexor function. It may therefore continue to act as a deforming force. The procedure does nothing to improve hip extension. The results of its use in children with spina bifida have been poor (Cruess & Turner 1970) and it can not be recommended.

Posterolateral iliopsoas transfer (Sharrard 1964)

This procedure is a modification of the Mustard iliopsoas transfer (Sharrard 1964). Instead of the tendon being transferred laterally to the greater trochanter it is moved posterolaterally though a hole in the iliac bone. By this means, as well as removing the principal deforming force, it is hoped that, in its new posterolateral position it will act to reinforce both abduction and extension, thereby restoring muscle balance. The procedure is indicated where imbalance between the adductors and flexors on one hand and the abductors and extensors on the other produces subluxation or dislocation in a child who has good walking potential. If performed early enough it may be effective in preventing the development of dysplasia and, in these circumstances, may be the only procedure required. If, however, the hip has already been dislocated or there has been marked subluxation, then the capsule will indubitably have been stretched and it would seem prudent to perform reefing of the capsule as part of the procedure. If the acetabulum is dysplastic reconstruction, either in the form of acetabuloplasty or pelvic osteotomy, is also indicated.

The method of transfer has been well described by Sharrard (1964) and is

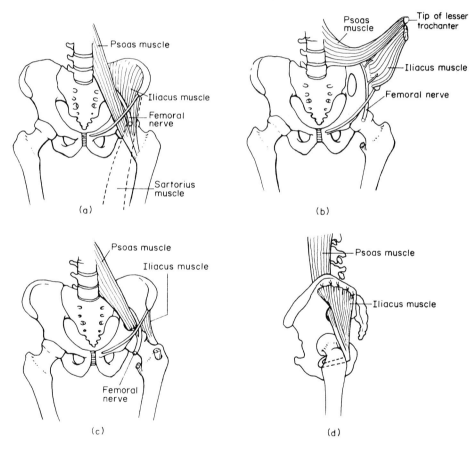

Fig. 10.9 Sharrard iliopsoas transfer — operative technique. (a) The normal anatomy of the operative field. (b) After detachment of the lesser trochanter complete mobilization of the iliacus and formation of a foramen lateral to the sacroiliac joint. (c) Anterior view after transplantation of the iliopsoas tendon to the posterolateral aspect of the greater trochanter. (d) Lateral view to show the iliacus lying on the outer side of the ilium. (From Sharrard W. J. W. (1971) *Paediatric Orthopaedics and Fractures,* Blackwell Scientific Publications, Oxford).

illustrated in his figure (Fig. 10.9) reproduced here. The reader is referred to this original article for operative details. Prior to the transfer being done an adductor release may be required as around 60° abduction is necessary to allow proper fixation of the iliopsoas to the trochanter. Instead of detaching the iliopsoas from the lesser trochanter from above, as described in Sharrard's account, we prefer to detach it via a medial incision. The trochanter is exposed as described previously and, using a curved on the flat osteotome, it is detached along with the attached iliopsoas. Later in the procedure when the femoral nerve has been exposed, it it retracted medially and the lesser trochanter is passed up from the groin wound using Kocher forceps.

The results and effectiveness of the procedure are not easy to evaluate. In particular lack of comparibility between various series and the use of additional procedures makes the interpretation of the available data very difficult. Suffice to say that, despite having been performed for over twenty years, it is still uncertain whether the results of transferring the iliopsoas are superior to those obtained by simply dividing it (Menelaus 1980). Attempts to judge the operation's effectiveness have been made by measuring its effect on hip stability, the resolution of bony deformity produced, on the child's gait and bracing requirements and by direct recording of the activity in the transferred muscle.

Stability as judged by the radiographic position of the femoral head is easiest of these parameters to study (Fig. 10.10), yet, even here, there are wide variations in the reported results.Thus while Jackson *et al.* (1979) found that, of those hips which were unstable preoperatively, only 30% achieved stability as a result of the procedure, Weisl and Mathews (1973) using the same criteria found 45% to be reduced. Parker and Walker (1975) reported an improvement in stability from 49% to 94%. More recently Bunch and Hakala (1984) reported successful reduction and its maintenance in 9 hips which were dislocated preoperatively. Other series have been reported by Menelaus (1980) and Carroll and Sharrard (1972).

The effect of the operation on a child's gait would appear to depend on the muscle power present preoperatively. Thus Sharrard (1964) found that, if there were no active abduction present the child would still have a Trendelenberg gait postoperatively, whereas, if there were some activity present then they might attain an almost normal gait.

The function of the transplanted muscle has been studied electromyographically by Buisson and Hamblen (1972). In their 16 patients electrical activity in the transplanted muscle was found in extension of the hip in only 3, whereas all but one showed activity on flexing the hip. They concluded that contraction of the iliopsoas held the hip in joint when flexion and adduction would normally tend to produce dislocation. Clinically function is more often found in abduction than in extension. Sharrard (1964) stated that if there were no active abduction or extension preoperatively, then voluntary abduction might be found in 40% postoperatively, but that active extension was seldom found. These results are in broad agreement with those of later investigators (Lee & Carroll 1985, Sherk &

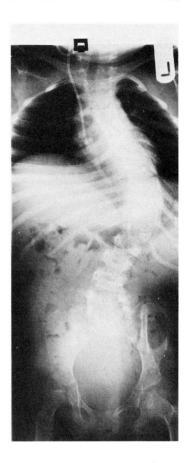

Fig. 10.10 After Sharrard iliopsoas transfer. Hip reduction has been maintained and the pelvis is level.

Ames 1978, Stillwell & Menelaus 1983, Carroll & Sharrard 1972, Weisl & Mathews 1973).

Obviously the other effect of transferring the iliopsoas is that its flexor activity is lost. Critics of the procedure feel that this loss of flexor power may produce increased disability (McKay *et al.* 1976). On the other hand, its proponents suggest otherwise. Menelaus for example felt that loss of flexor power was less disabling than the persistence of a fixed flexion deformity. Lee and Carroll (1965) estimated loss of flexor power to be around 1 MRC grade. Obviously the main importance of the loss is its functional effect. Stillwell and Menelaus (1983) found this to be minimal. Of the 47 patients they studied none appeared to have decreased walking capabilities and all but 3 could go up and down stairs inferring at least adequate flexor power. Benton *et al.* (1975) reported similar findings.

The rate and range of complications are not inconsiderable and are a common theme running through all reported series. Carroll and Sharrard (1972) reported stiffness, such that flexion past 90° was impossible, in 19 of 58 hips. Parker and Walker (1975), however, found only 1 stiff hip out of 72 operated on, and that due to ectopic bone formation. Fixed external rotation (Carroll & Sharrard 1972, Weisl

& Mathews 1973) or abduction (Menelaus 1980) is certainly a not uncommon complication but, unless extreme, may be of little functional importance. Avascular necrosis and fractures complicate a significant proportion of operations. The avascular necrosis rate varies from 10 to 25% (Carroll & Sharrard 1972, Rueda & Carroll 1972, Parker & Walker 1975) and is possibly due to residual adductor tightness. Fractures are even more common, the reported incidence varying from 20 to 50% (Freehafer et al. 1972, Rueda & Carroll 1972, Parker & Walker 1975).

All this merely emphasizes that the procedure should be undertaken only where substantial benefits can be aniticipated from a successful outcome.

Other muscle transfers

Several transfers, other than those of iliopsoas have been described. Some of these, for example, transfer of the fascia lata to erector spinae, have proven to be ineffective when used in myelomeningocele (Hogshead & Ponseti 1964, Basset et al. 1982). Transfer of the external oblique aponeurosis to the greater trochanter (Yngve & Lindseth 1982) and the adductor origin to the ischium (McKay et al. 1976) have shown promising results, but whether they will ultimately prove more effective than transfers involving the iliopsoas must await futher evaluation.

Bony procedures

Acetabuloplasty

Acetabular reconstruction is indicated when, in addition to subluxation or dislocation, dysplasia is present. Then, it is usually combined with a procedure aimed at achieving muscle balance. A prerequisite for its performance is an adequate sized acetabulum. If this is not the case, as for example might be found when the hip has been dislocated from birth, an alternative method of obtaining femoral head cover, such as the Chiari osteotomy, should be used (Lee & Carroll 1985).

The Pemberton acetabuloplasty is perhaps the most widely used. In this procedure the hip is exposed via a Smith–Peterson approach. The iliac apophysis is split and the muscles on both the medial and lateral sides of the iliac bone reflected subperiosteally until the sciatic notch can be easily palpated. The hip capsule is then exposed on the lateral side. Any capsule that is superiorly adherent to the iliac bone above its true level should be reflected back to its attachment using a periosteal elevator. If, as is almost invariably the case, the hip has been dislocated, the capsule should be opened preparatory to a capsulorrhaphy. This has the advantage of allowing the level of the osteotomy to be judged with some accuracy. With retractors in the sciatic notch each table of the ilium is osteotomized separately. The level of the osteotomy should be just above the capsular insertion and the direction follows that of the acetabulum. Using a curved on the flat osteotome, once over the dome of the acetabulum it should be directed down anteriorly to the sciatic notch such that the osteotomy terminates in the ilioischial limb of the triradiate cartilage rather than in the sciatic notch. A similarly directed osteotomy is then made in the other table of the ilium. The roof of the acetabulum can then be lowered over the femoral head to the required degree by inserting an osteotome and levering it down. A wedge of bone, taken from the anterior part of iliac crest, is inserted between the osteotomized surfaces. Hip reduction is then checked and repair of the capsule performed. If necessary this may be followed by an iliopsoas transfer. Six weeks in a hip spica is sufficient postoperative immobilization.

Chiari osteotomy

The Chiari osteotomy is preferable to acetabuloplasty under two circumstances: when, due to congenital dislocation, the acetabulum is small and poorly developed, and in the older child. Whilst it may need to be combined with muscle balancing procedures, if any abductor power is present, this will be augmented by the displacement of the osteotomy (Canale *et al.* 1975). The same author has reported excellent results with the use of the procedure, both in terms of hip stability and improved mobility.

Salter osteotomy

There is seldom any place for this procedure in the myelomeningocele hip. The maldirection of the acetabulum, typically found in congenital dislocation of the hip and which this operation is designed to correct, is simply not present. Instead, the acetabulum is circumferentially deficient so that altering its direction merely produces a secondary deficiency elsewhere.

Femoral osteotomy

The place of femoral osteotomy is not well established for two reasons. Firstly, in the presence of muscle imbalance, bony procedures performed in isolation will have at best a temporary effect. Secondly, because of reduced muscle activity around the hip, the potential for acetabular remodelling, even when the hip is correctly located, is very limited. Without doubt muscle imbalance around the hip leads to the development of anteversion and coxa valga. The converse, however, is true and resolution of the deformities can be expected if balance is restored, for example by posterolateral iliopsoas transfer (Freehafer *et al.* 1972). Only a temporary effect can be anticipated if femoral osteotomy alone is performed and the proximal femoral bony deformity will recur (McKay 1976) as will redislocation. In general it is felt that proximal femoral bony deformities are incidental and do not require treatment *per se* (Cruess & Turner 1970, Menelaus 1980).

Hip stiffness

Hip stiffness may follow any operation around the hip in the child with myelomeningocele. It is particularly common though after intra-articular procedures (Fig. 10.11). Treatment is difficult. Resection of the proximal femur may seem an obvious solution but the results of this have been unpredictable. Taylor (1985) in a series of 12 hips found that 8 were ankylosed at follow-up and 10 of the 12 showed extensive new bone formation. Fiewell (1978) on the other hand seems to have avoided this complication by the use of 90/90 traction for four weeks, all 13 of his patients maintaining flexion. The complication of ectopic bone formation is much more commonly found in paraplegia, whatever its cause. As new bone formation is never found above the level of the paralysis, it will be appreciated that it is almost exclusively found in children with thoracic neurosegmental levels. As they will be wheelchairbound such loss of flexion as a result of ectopic calcification has disastrous consequences and may present almost insoluble seating problems.

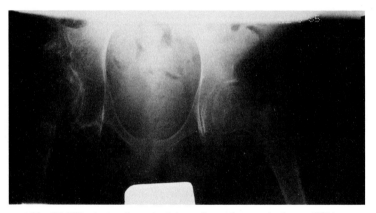

Fig. 10.11 Postoperative ectopic bone formation producing a stiff hip.

Cerebral palsy

Definition

Cerebral palsy is a nonprogressive brain disorder occuring before or during birth, or during the first years of life. It is characterized by poor development of postural reflexes and the retention of primitive patterns of activity. There is invariably a delay of normal motor development and reduced voluntary muscle function.

Disturbance of the central nervous system may involve different parts of the brain, which in turn produces different types of motor abnormality:

Spasticity

Dysfunction of the pyramidal system allows exaggeration of the spinal stretch reflex when inhibitory cortical control is reduced. There is increased muscle tone, particularly in the upper extremity flexors and the lower limb extensors. Patterns of voluntary movement are decreased because of facilitation of certain muscle groups, for example the hip adductors, combined with a relative inhibition of the abductors. Contractures appear early due to the persistent posturing of joints within a limited range of movement. This pattern of motor disorder can lead to progressive subluxation and dislocation of the hip (Fig. 10.12).

Motion disorder (dyskinesia)

This results from damage to the extrapyramidal system. It produces reduced muscle tone, poor control of posture, and is sometimes associated with abnormal involuntary movements, which are present only when the patient is awake. Contractures develop late and may be related more to persistent abnormal positioning of the child than to imbalance of muscle groups. One particular pattern of abnormality included in this group is called dystonia, or tension athetosis. This can mimic spasticity, but relaxation of the patient or repeated rapid movement, such as shaking a limb, results in decreased tone. Failure to recognize this small group of patients can lead to iatrogenic contractures. For example, surgical release of the adductors will result in wide fixed abduction of the hip.

Mixed

This represents a mixture of the first two types. All three forms may have asymmetry of involvement.

Distribution of motor disorder

The ability to walk, and the effect on the hip joint, also depends on the distribution of the motor disorder. Three classical patterns are described:

Hemiplegia

This involves one side of the body. Motor development is delayed but all the patients are able to walk, on average aged 21 months.

Diplegia

Spastic involvement of both lower limbs becomes evident at about six months of age and walking may be delayed until as late as 8 years. The spastic involvement is greater in the lower limbs, with minor involvement of the hands and arms. It may be associated with increased femoral anteversion and an internally rotated position of the leg while walking. Hip adduction and flexion contractures may also develop.

Quadriplegia

All four limbs are involved, and as a result head and trunk control is usually poor. The majority of these patients are confined to a wheelchair. Hip dislocation and scoliosis are most common in this group of patients, and interfere further with the ability to sit independently.

Management of the hip

During the assessment and treatment of cerebral palsy the hip cannot be taken in isolation. For example, in the quadriplegic patient, hip deformity is frequently associated with pelvic obliquity and scoliosis. In the diplegic patient the posture of the hip may be part of a flexor or extensor pattern affecting the whole of the lower limb. Surgical treatment of the hip has therefore on occasions to be undertaken in combination with operations on the knee and ankle. While this chapter inevitably focuses on the problems of the hip joint, its involvement as part of a total disturbance of motor control should not be forgotten. The problems affecting the hip in the chairbound spastic quadriplegic and in the walking patient are different, although there is some overlap. The natural history of the disability and treatment of the hip is therefore presented according to these clinical categories.

Chairbound child

Windswept deformity
This problem usually occurs in spastic quadriplegia. During the first six months of life the hip musculature is hypotonic, but from six months onwards spasticity of the hip adductors and flexors becomes detectable. It is important, as mentioned above, to differentiate between spasticity and dystonia. Rigidity also differs from spasticity in that the resistance to hip abduction occurs throughout the range of

movement, and the limb tends to remain in abduction rather than spring back into an adducted position when the examiners hands are removed. By two years of age there is usually a restricted range of hip abduction, associated with the hip flexion contracture. Letts *et al.* (1984) have studied the sequence of events and found that by three years of age almost half of the patients in this category had subluxation of one hip. The restriction of abduction was worse on the subluxed side. The great majority also had tight adductors on the opposite side, but a small minority exhibited an abduction contracture on the side of the stable hip. The femoral head lateralizes progressively, and the average age at dislocation was seven years. The acetabular index, which is a measure of abnormal growth, only increased after the onset of subluxation, indicating that this is the result rather than the cause of the subluxation. The most common temporal sequence was that the dislocation was followed by pelvic obliquity, and finally scoliosis (Fig. 10.12).

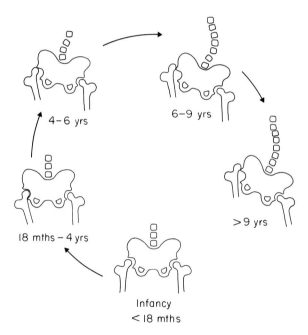

4–6 yrs

6–9 yrs

>9 yrs

18 mths – 4 yrs

Infancy
< 18 mths

Fig. 10.12 The genesis of the windswept hip phenomenon.
(Redrawn with permission from Letts *et al.* 1984).

This sequence of events results in a deformity of the body sometimes called a windswept syndrome. One hip is adducted, flexed and internally rotated, whereas the other is in relative abduction and external rotation. The high side of the oblique pelvis is on the side of the adducted hip, and it is probable that the spasticity and contracture of the iliopsoas and hip adductors are responsible for the progressive subluxation of the femoral head (Fig. 10.13a). It is interesting that the high side of the pelvis and convexity of the scoliosis are on the opposite side in the great majority of the patients, although this is not always so. The effect of the adduction

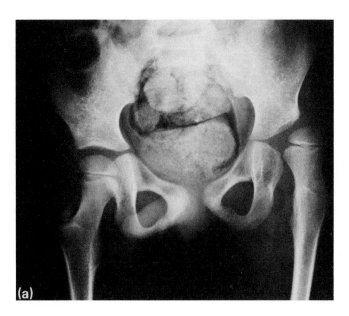

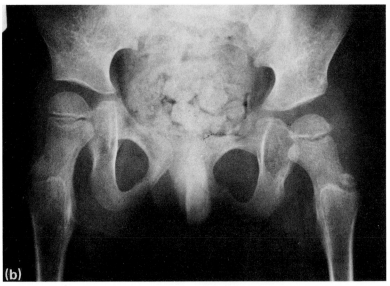

Fig. 10.13 (a) The radiograph of a seven-year-old chairbound spastic quadriplegic, with subluxation of the left femoral head.
(b) One year after bilateral adductor release and anterior obturator neurectomy.

deformity is different when sitting or standing. An adducted hip which produces a short leg when standing, produces rotation of the pelvis from the coronal plane while sitting (Fig. 10.14). Rotational deformity at the hip produces pelvic obliquity and scoliosis when sitting. (Rang *et al.* 1981).

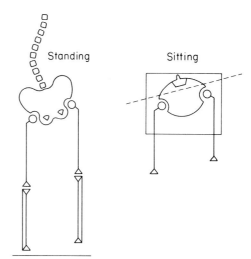

Standing   Sitting

Fig. 10.14 An adduction
contracture while standing
produces apparent shortening of
the leg, but while sitting produces
pelvic rotation. (Redrawn with
permission from Rang *et al.*
1981.)

Treatment

The objective is to maintain a good sitting posture, with or without external support.
The development of infrapelvic contractures and hip dislocation makes this more
difficult. It is best to maintain a straight spine and level pelvis by preventing the
development of the windswept posture rather than trying to treat the frankly
dislocated femoral head and its associated secondary deformities. Clinical screening
should start at the latest by two years of age, and an annual hip radiograph is
recommended.

Position of the hip

A daily therapy programme, beginning in infancy, is beneficial but is usually not
effective alone. Persistent positioning of the child in the same lateral sleeping
posture can precipitate asymmetry of posture during the first year of life even in
normal children. It is therefore important that, if the lateral position is used for
sleeping, the baby should be placed on alternate sides (Fulford & Brown 1976).
Night splinting is particularly helpful in removing excessive stretch from weaker
muscles, such as the hip abductors. Small children will accept trunk and lower
extremity abduction orthoses but older children do not tolerate this degree of
control (Drennan 1983). Abduction seating or a pommel seat also ensure continued
abduction of the hips during the day.

Prophylactic surgery

If despite these measures the total range of hip abduction becomes less than 20°

or there is early radiological subluxation of the femoral head, prophylactic surgical treatment may be indicated. Bilateral adductor release and anterior obturator neurectomy is undertaken in the majority of cases (Fig. 10.13). If a hip flexion contracture is also present, the iliopsoas is also released. Following soft tissue surgery the child is kept in abduction in broomstick plasters for three weeks. Continued abduction seating or night splinting is then essential.

In the occasional case with a contralateral abduction contracture, a unilateral adductor release may be indicated. Under these circumstances careful follow-up is required as the unoperated hip may occasionally develop an adduction deformity and subluxate within a year.

With this programme of early detection of hips at risk and appropriate soft tissue surgery, it is hoped to avoid bony surgery such as femoral varus osteotomy.

Surgery for dislocation

In the older child the problem of progressive dislocation and acetabular dysplasia becomes increasingly difficult to treat. The authors' preference for nonambulant children in these circumstances has been to undertake radical soft tissue surgery to minimize or correct a fixed infrapelvic deformity, but not to undertake bony surgery to relocate or cover the femoral head. It is not the dislocation which causes pelvic obliquity and rotation, but the associated contractures.

If the hip is dislocated with a flexion–adduction deformity, then the appropriate releases and posterolateral transfer of the iliopsoas can maintain the reduction in most cases (Sharrard 1980). Excessive tension of the transfer should be avoided as it results in limited hip flexion, with difficulty in sitting.

However, Hoffer *et al.* (1985) suggest that if, after effective soft tissue releases, the femoral head remains subluxated because of excessive valgus angulation, anteversion, or both, a varus derotation osteotomy of the femur should be performed. However, they found that despite reduction of the hip for long periods, acetabular remodelling did not occur.

Many of the children seen late with established dislocation and scoliosis have such severe brain damage that is seems both kinder and wiser to ignore their deformities. Functional gains have been minimal, the risks of anaethesia and surgery considerable, and the child would be subjected to discomfort. Unfortunately, an established dislocation in a young adult can sometimes be associated with troublesome pain. Frequently the patient is unable to communicate verbally, but appears to be in pain when the hip is moved for example while being dressed. Although a modified Girdlestone arthroplasty has been advocated in this situation (Castle & Schneider 1978), in the authors' experience it may still be associated with spasm and pain around the hip. Total hip replacement is not recommended for the dislocated hip which is part of a wind-swept deformity. A painful subluxated hip can be helped by release of contractures and a pelvic osteotomy using the principle described by Chiari (1974). Arthrodesis is recommended for the frank dislocation which produces distressing pain (Root 1983). The hip should be fused in 45° flexion, 15° of abduction and neutral rotation.

Slouched deformity

An alternative pattern of sitting posture which may develop is associated with hamstring spasticity and contracture. The short hamstrings prevent the hip from flexing adequately, which results in the pelvis being tilted backwards and the child sitting in a slouched position of spinal flexion. Later, fixed knee flexion contractures and a fixed thoracic kyphosis develop (Fig. 10.15). Unlike the windswept posture, the hamsting tightness is usually symmetrical.

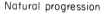

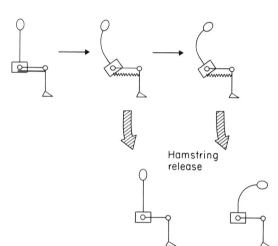

Fig. 10.15 Hamstring shortening produces backward tilt of the pelvis and compensatory spinal flexion, which can be corrected by early release. Untreated, a progressive dorsal kyphosis develops, and late release leaves the child looking downwards. (Redrawn with permission from Rang *et al.* 1981.)

Minor contracture of the hamstrings can be compensated while sitting by increasing knee flexion. This can be provided by raising the front edge of the chair with a four inch wedge. This flexes the hips and knees, and also stops the child from sliding forwards. However, patients who cannot flex the hip to a right angle without excessive knee flexion, require hamstring lengthening. This is undertaken proximally through a medial approach (Bell 1973). This can more than double straight leg raising and improves the sitting posture (Rang *et al.* 1981).This procedure is contraindicated in the older child when a fixed thoracic kyphosis has developed, because, when the pelvis is in the corrected position, the upper trunk will be leaning forwards and the face looking downwards (Fig. 10.15).

Rarely, a severe extension–abduction contracture can develop. This is most likely to occur in patients with athetosis or rigidity, either spontaneously or following adductor releases. It causes major difficulties in obtaining a satisfactory sitting position. As well as proximal hamstring release, the gluteus maximus insertion and external rotators may need division. The sciatic nerve may be under considerable tension when the hip is then flexed to a right angle, and decompression by femoral shortening may be required (Szalay *et al.* 1986).

The walking child

The onset of walking is delayed, and some children may develop a limited ability even as late as 8 years of age. It is helpful to be able to make a clinical assessment as early as possible as to whether a child is likely to walk. In this respect Bleck (1975) has provided guidelines based upon the presence or absence of infantile reflexes, at one year of age. This will allow the goals of treatment to be defined in relation to whether the child is likely to walk or be confined to a wheelchair. Early orthopaedic surgery designed to improve function may actually delay the onset of walking in spastic diplegia. It is therefore better to defer surgery on children who have a good prognosis but are not yet walking, until a walking pattern has been established. The exception to this general rule applies to the development of progressive adduction contractures and subluxation of the femoral head.

The whole child and not only the hips must be examined. The child should be examined on a couch to elicit the presence of hip and knee flexion contractures, and tightness of the hip adductors and hamstrings. Equinus contracture can be assessed both with the knee extended and flexed to a right angle. These physical signs, which measure shortening of muscles in a lower motor neuron disorder, may be misleading when applied to cerebral palsy. Perry *et al.* (1976) found the stretch tests to be non-specific, and in this respect found electromyography helpful in determining which muscle groups are overactive. Such studies are undertaken when the child is walking, as part of a gait assessment. The recent technical developments in gait analysis allow the surgeon to plan treatment and to evaluate the result with more objective criteria (Perry *et al.* 1976, Sutherland 1978, Gage *et al.* 1984). A sophisticated gait laboratory is extremely expensive to fund, and not available for all patients. However, some assessment of the functional benefit of treatment can be made with equipment as simple as a stopwatch and a measured walkway (Butler *et al.* 1984). Using gait analysis we have found that on occasions surgical treatment has improved both the appearance of the patient's walking and the energy consumption. On other occasions the appearance may have improved but at the expense of an increased energy cost.

With regards to the hip, the development of an adduction, flexion and internal rotation posture may occur individually or in any combination.

Adduction deformity

Spasticity of the adductors produces a narrow based, or scissoring gait associated with a short stride length. It is generally agreed that tenotomy should be undertaken when hip abduction is limited to 20° or less, with or without the presence of scissoring. It is usual to do an adductor release without an anterior obturator neurectomy in the walking child. It has been suggested that adductor myotomy associated with obturator neurectomy is indicated for scissoring gait (Banks & Green 1960), but there is probably no significant long term advantage with a neurectomy as long as the contracture has been corrected. Even more important than the details of the operation is the postoperative care, which applies the principle of maintaining wide abduction until the lengthening of the adductors is established permanently. Postoperatively the legs are held abducted in a broomstick cast for three weeks and this then being replaced by an abduction night splint. A physiotherapy programme concentrates on strengthening the abductors and developing a balanced walking pattern (Banks & Green 1960).

An alternative procedure is transfer of the adductors origin to the ischium, which converts the muscle from an accessory hip flexor to an extensor. It has been claimed that this gives better results, both early and late, than adductor tenotomy with or without neurectomy (Root & Spero 1981). The transferred muscle apparently provides greater pelvic stability, decreases hip flexion contracture, and reduces instability of the hip. However, this is at the expense of a longer surgical procedure and a higher incidence of postoperative complications. There is no difference in the radiographic benefit of the two procedures with regard to lateral migration of the femoral head (Schultz et al. 1984), and this technically demanding procedure probably has limited application for most patients with cerebral palsy.

Flexion deformity

Flexion deformity at the hip while standing and walking may be associated with a varying degree of internal rotation. The positions of the knees and ankles are variable, and in the young child depend on the postural control of the limbs by the damaged brain. With increased age, secondary shortening or contracture of muscle groups may occur. It is important not to consider the hip in isolation, but to plan the most appropriate treatment for the whole limb which can be undertaken at one intervention.

In addition to performing the Thomas test, the flexion deformity can be measured clinically with the patient lying prone (Fig. 10.6) (Staheli 1977). A static measurement while standing has been described by Bleck (1971) by taking a lateral radiograph of the sacrum and femur on the same exposure. Lines are drawn across the superior surface of the sacrum and along the axis of the femur (Fig. 10.16). They bisect to form the sacrofemoral angle. Severity of hip flexion deformity can also be measured while walking in the gait laboratory.

Weakening of the spastic hip flexors by recession of the iliopsoas is advocated for a clinical hip flexion deformity in excess of 20° or a sacrofemoral angle less than 45° (Bleck 1980). If the knees are hyperextended, an additional release of the rectus femoris is indicated. Alternatively, if the knees are flexed due to spastic hamstrings, it is usual to perform additional distal lengthening of the hamstrings. The combined hip and knee flexor release will improve extension of the limb during the stance

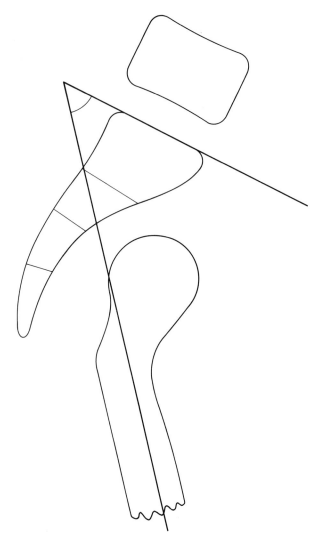

Fig. 10.16 Measurement of the
sacrofemoral angle on a standing
lateral radiograph.

phase of gait, but sometimes the knee will not flex freely during swing phase. As
a result the foot drags along the floor, thus increasing the energy expenditure and
making it almost impossible for the patient to walk up steps. The recent recognition
of cospasticity of the hamstrings and quadriceps, has allowed a distal rectus femoris
release or transfer to be performed at the same time. This achieves an improvement
of the swing as well as the stance phase of gait (Gage *et al.* 1986). The selection of
patients for such surgery is assisted greatly by the facility to demonstrate abnormal
electromyographic activity of the rectus femoris muscle while the patient is walking.

Internal rotation deformity

Occasionally, there is a marked internal rotation deformity at the hip which presents with the feet turned inwards and a laborious, weaving gait due to restricted pelvic rotation. This is associated with excessive internal femoral torsion. According to Bleck (1980) there is acceptable functional correction of this gait in the majority of young patients by soft tissue surgery alone. He advocates a recession of the iliopsoas from the lesser trochanter to the anterior capsule of the hip. In older children, over 8 years of age, derotation osteotomy of the femur is also required. A completely different surgical approach for this problem has been advocated by Steel (1980). The gluteus medius and minimus insertions are transferred from the greater trochanter to the anterior part of the femur to change their function from that of inward rotators to that of outward rotators. It is reported as being a satisfactory procedure, but does sacrifice abduction strength in approximately 10% of patients.

Hip subluxation

Prevention is possible and should be the goal of treatment. It is only after the femoral head has begun to sublux that acetabular dysplasia occurs. The management consists of early recognition by periodic clinical examination and radiographs, with soft tissue surgery for a range of adduction of 20° or less. Unfortunately in some patients subluxation can occur in the absence of adductor spasticity or contracture. Subluxation in the child with a good prognosis for walking can usually be resolved by soft tissue surgery. This consists of iliopsoas recession (Bleck 1971), with adductor release if abduction is restricted. It is probable that, once a child has started walking, additional bony surgery will resolve the problem with more certainty. A femoral

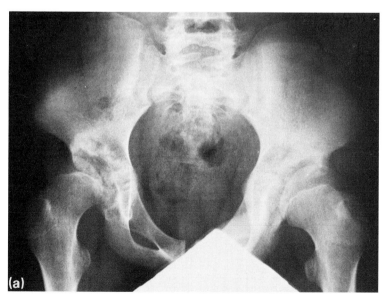

Fig. 10.17 (a) The radiograph of a 13-year-old boy, able to walk, shows subluxation of the hips and a break in Shenton's line on the right.

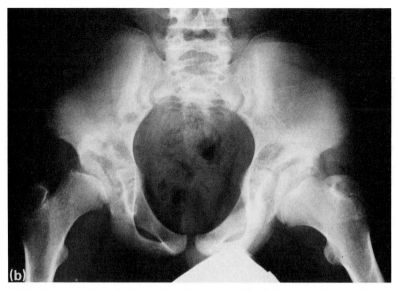

Fig. 10.17 (b) The position of the right femoral head is improved by abduction and internal rotation of the leg. This position can be maintained by a varus derotation osteotomy of the femur.

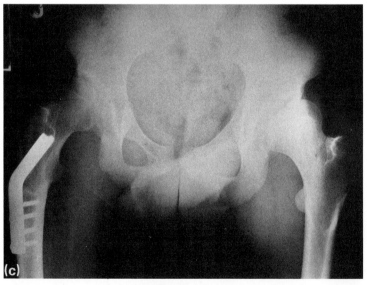

Fig. 10.17 (c) At skeletal maturity, three years after the osteotomy, Shenton's line remains intact. The acetabular dysplasia has not improved.

osteotomy is indicated for a reduceable subluxation (Fig. 10.17; Hoffer *et al.* 1985). Abduction of 45° is a prerequisite and an osteotomy is usually therefore preceded by an adductor release. Following this a radiograph of the hip in abduction on the operating table will show whether the subluxation has been reduced. If it is satisfactory a varus osteotomy may be performed, reducing the neck shaft angle to between 110° and 120°. Less than this will produce excessive abductor weakness, and shortening of the limb. Excessive anteversion is corrected by external rotation of the femoral shaft, planning to retain 20° only of the internal rotation at the hip.

If the head does not reduce fully into the acetabulum, acetabular augmentation is indicated. This can be achieved by a pelvic osteotomy, using the principle described by Chiari (1974). The authors prefer the transtrochanteric approach

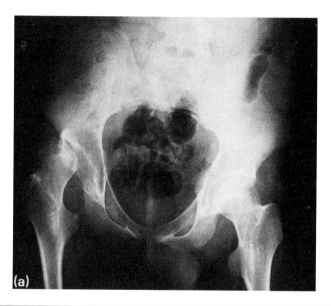

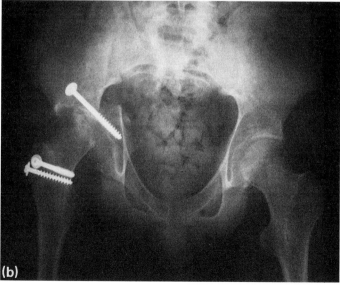

Fig. 10.18 (a) The radiograph of a 17-year-old boy, complaining of pain in the right hip while walking. (b) One year after adductor release and pelvic osteotomy, using the transtrochanteric approach, the hip is pain free.

(Kawamura *et al.* 1982), and fix the osteotomy with a cancellous lag screw in order to avoid a plaster cast and to allow immediate postoperative mobilization of the patient (Fig. 10.18). A shelf procedure has also been described for this purpose (Zuckerman *et al.* 1984).

References

Asher M. & Olson J. (1983) Factors affecting ambulatory status of patients with spina bifida cystica. *Journal of Bone and Joint Surgery,* **65A,** 350–6.

Banks H. H. & Green W. T. (1960) Adductor myotomy and obturator neurectomy for the correction of adduction contracture of the hip in cerebral palsy. *Journal of Bone and Joint Surgery,* **42A,** 111–26.

Bassett G., Weinstein S. & Cooper R. (1982) Long-term follow-up of fascia lata transfer for the paralytic hip in myelodysplasia. *Journal of Bone and Joint Surgery,* **64A,** 360–5.

Bell M. (1973) Proximal hamsting release — anterior approach. *Journal of Bone and Joint Surgery,* **55B,** 661.

Benton I. J., Salvati E. A. & Root L. (1975) Reconstructive surgery in the myelomeningocele hip. *Clinical Orthopedics and Related Research,* **110,** 261–8.

Bleck E. E. (1971) Postural and gait abnormalities caused by hip-flexion deformity in spastic cerebral palsy. *Journal of Bone and Joint Surgery,* **53A,** 1468–88.

Bleck E. E. (1975) Locomotor prognosis in cerebral palsy. *Developmental Medicine and Child Neurology,* **17,** 18–25.

Bleck E. E. (1980) The hip in cerebral palsy. *Orthopaedic Clinics of North America,* **11,** 79–104.

Buisson J. S. & Hamblen D. L. (1972) Electromyographic assessment of the transplanted iliopsoas muscle in spina bifida cystica. *Developmental Medicine and Child Neurology,* Supp. **27,** 29–33.

Bunch W. H. & Hakala M. W. (1984) Iliopsoas transfer in children with myelomeningocele. *Journal of Bone and Joint Surgery,* **66A,** 224–227.

Butler P., Engelbrecht M., Major R. E., Tait J. H., Stallard J. & Patrick J. H. (1984) Physiological cost index of walking for normal children and its use as an indicator of physical handicap. *Developmental Medicine and Child Neurology,* **26,** 607–12.

Canale T. S., Hammond N. L., Cotler J. M. & Sneddon H. E. (1975) Pelvic displacement osteotomy for chronic hip dislocation in myelomeningocele. *Journal of Bone and Joint Surgery,* **57A,** 177–83.

Carroll N. & Sharrard W. J. W. (1972) Long term follow-up of posterior iliopsoas transplantation for paralytic dislocation of the hip. *Journal of Bone and Joint Surgery,* **54A,** 551–60.

Castle M. E. & Schneider C. (1978) Proximal femoral resection — interposition arthroplasty. *Journal of Bone and Joint Surgery,* **60A,** 1051–4.

Chiari K. (1974) Medial displacement osteotomy of the pelvis. *Clinical Orthopaedics,* **98,** 55–71.

Cruess R. L. & Turner N. S. (1970) Paralysis of the hip abductor muscles in spina bifida. *Journal of Bone and Joint Surgery,* **52A,** 1364–72.

Dias L. S. (1983) In Schafer M. F. & Dias L. S. (eds.) *Myelomingocele Orthopaedic Treatment.* Williams and Wilkins, Baltimore.

Drennan J. C. (1983) *Orthopaedic Management of Neuromuscular Disorders,* pp. 231–237, p. 262. J. B. Lippincott, Philadelphia.

Erken E. H. W. (1984) The hip in myelomeningocele. *Journal of Bone and Joint Surgery,* **66B,** 451.

Feiwell E. Sakai D. & Blatt T. (1978) The effect of hip reduction on function in patients with myelomeningocele. *Journal of Bone and Joint Surgery,* **60A,** 169–73.

Freehafer A. A., Vessely J. C. & Malk R. P. (1972) Iliopsoas muscle transfer in the treatment of myelomeningocele patients with paralytic hip deformities. *Journal of Bone and Joint Surgery,* **54,** 1715–29.

Fulford G. E. & Brown J. K. (1976) Position as a cause of deformity in children with cerebral palsy. *Developmental Medicine and Child Neurology* **18,** 305–14.

Gage J. R., Fabian D., Hicks R. & Tashman S. (1984) Pre- and post-operative gait analysis in patients with spastic diplegia: a preliminary report. *Journal of Pediatric Orthopedics,* **4,** 715–25.

Gage J., Perry J., Hicks R. R., Koop S. & Werntz J. R. (1986) Rectus femoris transfer as a means of improving knee function in cerebral palsy. Presented to Pediatric Orthopedic Society of North America, Boston.

Hoffer, M. M., Stein G. A., Koffman M. & Prietto M. (1985) Femoral varus-derotation osteotomy in spastic cerebral palsy. *Journal of Bone and Joint Surgery,* **67A,** 1229–35.

Hogshead H. P. & Ponseti I. V. (1969) Fascia lata transfer to the erector spinae for the treatment of flexion abduction contractures of the hip in patients with poliomyelitis and myelomeningocele. *Journal of Bone and Joint Surgery,* **46A,** 1389–404.

Huff C. W. & Ramsay P. L. (1978) Myelodysplasia; the influence of the quadriceps and hip abductor muscles for ambulatory function and stabilization of the hips. *Journal of Bone and Joint Surgery,* **60A,** 432–43.

Jackson R., Padgett T. T. & Donovan M. (1979) Posterior iliopsoas muscle transfer in myelodysplasia. *Journal of Bone and Joint Surgery,* **61A,** 40–5.

Kawamura B., Hosono S. & Yokogushi K. (1982) Dome osteotomy of the pelvis. In Tachdjian M. O. (ed.) *Congenital Dislocation of the Hip,* pp. 609–23. Churchill Livingstone, New York, Edinburgh and Melbourne.

Lee E. H. & Carroll N. C. (1985) Hip stability and ambulatory status in myelomeningocele. *Journal of Paediatric Orthopaedics,* **5,** 522–7.

Letts M., Shapiro L., Mulder K. & Klassen O. (1984) The windblown hip syndrome in total body cerebral palsy. *Journal of Pediatric Orthopedics,* **4,** 55–62.

Lorber J. (1971) Results of treatment of myelomeningocele. An analysis of 524 unselected cases with special reference to possible selection for treatment. *Developmental Medicine and Child Neurology,* **13,** 279–303.

McKay D. W., Jackman K., Nanson S. S. & Eng G. (1976) McKay hip stabilization in myelomeningocele. *Developmental Medicine and Child Neurology,* Suppl. **37,** 168–9.

McKibben B. (1973) The use of splintage in the management of paralytic hip dislocations in spina bifida cystical. *Journal of Bone and Joint Surgery,* **55B,** 163–72.

Menelaus M. B. (1976) Orthopaedic management of children with myelomeningocele. A plea for realistic goals. *Developmental Medicine and Child Neurology,* Suppl. **37,** 3–11.

Menelaus M. B. (1980) *The Orthopaedic Mangement of Spina Bifida Cystica,* p. 28. Churchill Livingstone, Edinburgh.

Mustard W. T. (1959) A follow-up study of iliopsoas transfer for hip instability. *Journal of Bone and Joint Surgery,* **41B,** 289–98.

Parker B. & Walker G. (1975) Posterior psoas transfer and hip instability in lumbar myelomeningocele. *Journal of Bone and Joint Surgery,* **57B,** 53–8.

Perry J., Hoffer M. M., Antonelli D., Plut J., Lewis G. & Greenberg R. (1976) Electromyography before and after surgery for hip deformity in children with cerebral palsy. *Journal of Bone and Joint Surgery,* **58A,** 201–8.

Rang M., Douglas G., Bennet G. C. & Koreska J. (1981) Seating for children with cerebral palsy. *Journal of Pediatric Orthopedics,* **1,** 279–87.

Root L. & Spero C. R. (1981) Hip adductor transfer compared with adductor tenotomy in cerebral palsy. *Journal of Bone and Joint Surgery,* **63A,** 767–71.

Root L. quoted by Drennan J. C. (1983) *Orthopaedic Management of Neuromuscular Disorders,* p. 283. J. P. Lippincott Company, Philadelphia & Toronto.

Rueda J. & Carroll N. C. (1972) Hip instability in patients with myelomeningocele. *Journal of Bone and Joint Surgery,* **54B,** 422–31.

Schaffer M. F. & Dias L. S. (1983) *Myelomeningocele Orthopaedic Treatment,* Williams and Wilkins, Baltimore.

Schultz R. S., Chamberlain S. E. & Stevens P. M. (1984) Radiographic comparison of adductor procedures in cerebral palsied hips. *Journal of Pediatric Orthopedics,* **4,** 741–4.

Sharrard W. J. W. (1964) Posterior iliopsoas transplantation in the treatment of paralytic dislocation of the hip. *Journal of Bone and Joint Surgery,* **46B,** 426–444.

Sharrard W. J. W. (1971) *Paediatric Orthopaedics and Fractures.* Blackwell Scientific Publications, Oxford.

Sharrard W. J. W. (1980) Paralytic dislocation of the hip in cerebral palsy and the place of iliopsoas transplantation. *Journal of Bone and Joint Surgery,* **62B,** 278.

Sherk H. H. & Ames M. D. (1978) Functional results of iliopsoas transfer in myelomeningocele hip dislocation. *Clinical Orthopaedics and Related Research,* **137,** 181–6.

Staheli L. T. (1977) The prone hip extension test. *Clinical Orthopaedics,* **123,** 12–15.

Stark G. D. & Baker G. C. (1967) The Neurological involvement of the lower limbs in myelomeningocele. *Developmental Medicine and Child Neurology,* **9,** 732–44.

Steel H. H. (1980) Gluteus medius and minimus insertion advancement for correction of internal rotation gait in spastic cerebral palsy. *Journal of Bone and Joint Surgery,* **62A,** 919–27.

Stillwell A. & Menelaus M. B. (1985) Walking in mature patients with spina bifida. *Journal of Paediatric Orthopaedics,* **3,** 184–90.

Sutherland D. H. (1978) Gait analysis in cerebral palsy. *Developmental Medicine and Child Neurology,* **20,** 807–13.

Szalay E. A., Roach J. W., Houkom J. A., Wenger D. R. & Herring J. A. (1986) Extension-abduction contracture of the spastic hip. *Journal of Pediatric Orthopedics,* **6,** 1–6.

Taylor L. J. (1985) Excision of the proximal end of the femur for very stiff hips in myelomeningocele. *Journal of Bone and Joint Surgery,* **67B,** 147–8.

Weisl H. (1983) Coxa vara in spina bifida. *Journal of Bone and Joint Surgery,* **65B,** 128–33.

Weisl H. & Mathews J. P. (1973) Posterior iliopsoas transfer in the management of the hip in spina bifida. *Developmental Medicine and Child Neurology,* Supp. **29,** 100–5.

Yngve D. A. & Lindseth R. E. (1982) Effectiveness of muscle transfer in myelomeningocele hips measured by radiographic indices. *Journal of Paediatric Orthopaedics,* **2,** 121–125.

Zuckerman J. D., Staheli L. T. & McLaughlin J. F. (1984) Acetabular augmentation for progressive hip subluxation in cerebral palsy. *Journal of Pediatric Orthopedics,* **4,** 436–42.

11

Miscellaneous Disorders

G. C. BENNET

Torsional abnormalities

Femoral torsion refers to the angle between the axis of the femoral neck and that of the transcondylar plane of the distal femur. A variable degree of torsion is normally present but only when excessive is it considered pathological. Whilst such excessive torsion is known to be associated with a variety of conditions such as congenital dislocation of the hip and cerebral palsy, the following section refers only to its occurrence in otherwise normal children. What importance the subject has lies in its effect on foot direction when walking. Basically internal femoral torsion or anteversion will produce intoeing, and external torsion or retroversion out-toeing. That internal torsion does have this effect has been shown by its direct measurement. Using both ultrasound (Moulton & Upadhyay 1982) and conventional radiography (Fabry et al. 1973) on children with a unilateral intoe gait, increased anteversion was consistently found on the affected side. Such gait abnormalities have a significance out of all proportion to their medical importance chiefly because of their frequency. Scrutton and Robson (1968) found that 18% of an unselected series of otherwise normal children intoed on one side. In a similar study (MacSweeny 1971) an intoe gait was found in 13.6% of children whereas out-toeing occured in only 0.5%. Two-thirds of those who intoed had increased internal femoral torsion.

Whilst these minor deformities generate much parental concern, there is no evidence to suggest that they have any harmful effect. In a study of school children and adults (Staheli et al. 1977) no relationship was found between athletic performance and torsional abnormalities. Nor has any evidence been found to suggest that their presence has any connection with the later development of degenerative joint disease (Kling & Hensinger 1983). We are, therefore, considering a cosmetic defect.

As torsional 'abnormalities' are present in the neonate it is not unreasonable to ascribe them to intrauterine position. Prenatally the hips are flexed and laterally rotated. This produces the increased range of external rotation normally found in the newborn. The feet tend to be internally rotated so that internal tibial torsion is the rule. Spontaneous resolution of both usually takes place by the second year of life.

It should be remembered, however, that factors other than bony architecture may affect the range of motion. The angle of anteversion generally reduces with age. From a maximum of around 60° at 30 weeks' gestation (Somerville 1957) it averages 40° in the newborn child and 16° at age 16 (Kling & Hensinger 1983). This, however, produces an apparent paradox as, during the first 2 years of life, internal rotation is increasing whilst anteversion is decreasing. Something other than configuration of the femur must be responsible. The likeliest explanation is that the posterior capsule of the hip joint is contracted secondary to the intrauterine position and, only once these soft tissue contractures stretch, can the effect of anteversion on rotation manifest itself. Thus, the range of external rotation reduces from being twice that of internal rotation in the first six months of life to being slightly less by the age of three (Coon et al. 1975).

Postnatal posture too has been implicated in the later development of torsional abnormalities. Sleeping prone with the legs extended in internal or external rotation or sitting in the television squat or the tailor's position are all said to cause torsion of one sort or another. Yet, whether this is the cause or whether the position the child adopts is merely that of maximum comfort imposed by pre-existing torsional deformities is not known (Sharrard 1979).

The amount of anteversion present can be measured radiographically or inferred by clinical examination. Several radiographic methods have been described, all of which aim, by standard positioning of the limb, to allow either direct measurement from the X-ray film or calculation of the angle of anteversion from tables (Ryder & Crane 1953, Dunlap et al. 1953, Dunn 1952, Hubbard & Staheli 1972). These methods are accurate and reproducible. Ultrasound too has been used with good results (Moulton & Upadhyay 1982) although it appears to become progressively less accurate as the degree of anteversion increases (Phillips et al. 1985). Whilst computerized tomography can give a degree of accuracy in excess of either of these methods, its use cannot be justified, either in terms of expense or, more importantly, on safety grounds as the radiation dosage is much greater than that associated with conventional radiography. Whilst all these methods have had their place in the better understanding of the condition, there seems little reason to subject children to them routinely and they might best be restricted to that very small number of children in whom surgery is contemplated. Even then, the practical value of the information obtained is questionable.

Children with an intoe gait may be referred for orthopaedic consultation for a variety of reasons, the first and foremost of which is appearance. Such children tend to look clumsy, particularly when wearing heavy winter footwear and almost invariably their repeated falling, which is probably no more than in a normal child, is blamed on their gait. Before honing in on the torsional abnormality, one should exclude any neuromuscular disorder as being responsible for their supposed (or real) clumsiness. Once this has been done, the aim of the clinical examination is to determine what, if any, torsional deformities are present, where they are, and, if at more than one level, whether the cumulative effect is compensatory or additive. This is achieved by the use of the torsional profile (Staheli 1977) as previously described in Chapter 2. The foot progression angle gives an impression of the cosmetic defect. It may of course be normal in someone with combined internal femoral and external tibial torsion (Fig. 11.1). A normal value lies between + 10 and 20°. Hip rotation and the thigh foot angle are then measured and the foot inspected to exclude metatarsus adductus (Fig. 11.2). It should be emphasized that whilst this is a reasonably reproducible examination, there is, as with any clinical examination, a margin of error so that only repeated and large changes should be considered significant (Luchini & Stevens 1983).

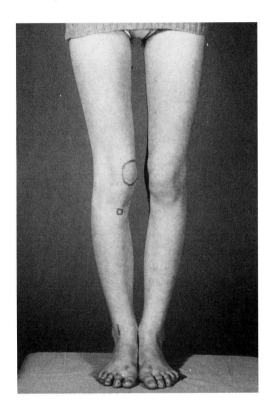

Fig. 11.1 Combined internal femoral and external tibial torsion. The patella, the tibial tubercle and a point on the ankle midway between the malleoli are marked. The tibial torsion compensates for the femoral torsion so that the foot progression angle is normal.

As the amount of anteversion present is related to the range of hip rotation, a clinical estimation of its severity can be obtained. Thus, mildly excessive internal femoral torsion is said to be present in a child with medial rotation of 70°–80° and lateral rotation of 10°–20° (2 or 3 SD from the mean), moderate when internal rotation is 80°–90° and external 0°–10 ° (3 to 4 SD from mean) whilst a severe case would be characterized by medial rotation of more than 90° and no external rotation (Staheli 1977).

The mere existance of excessive anteversion does not necessarily mean that

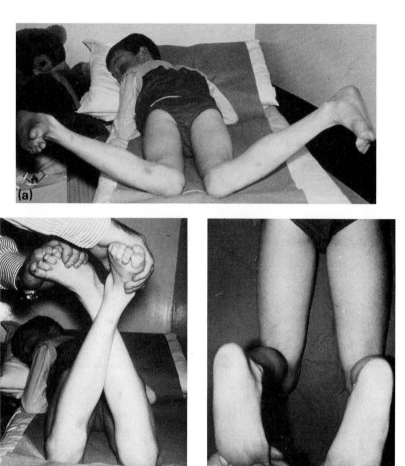

Fig. 11.2 The torsional profile of a boy with mild internal femoral torsion (hip internal rotation 70°, external rotation 15°) and internal tibial torsion (thigh foot angle −15°).

treatment is required. Sharrard (1979) found that half the children presenting with intoeing between the ages of 18 months and 3 years underwent spontaneous improvement such that, by the age of 5, the range of motion of the hip was normal. In those presenting after the age of three spontaneous correction was less certain whilst, after the age of 8, little could be anticipated. Management rather than treatment is indicated in this condition. It is very much easier to order useless, and often expensive, shoewear to satisfy the parents by making them feel that something is being done rather than taking time to explain the benign nature of the condition. Twisters, Denis-Browne splints and shoe modifications are still prescribed in spite of the fact that there is no evidence that such mechanical devices have any effect whatsoever on the natural history of the condition (Fabry *et al.* 1973, Staheli 1977, Kling & Hensinger 1983). Rather explanation, observation and the recording of clinical findings are the mainstay of management. Whilst it is current wisdom to advise parents to keep their children out of those sitting or lying positions which are thought to cause or perpetuate torsion, it may be that this too is of little value and that the child's position of rest will revert to normal spontaneously once the torsion has resolved. Femoral osteotomy is the only effective treatment for internal femoral torsion. Once equal internal and external hip rotation has been obtained by this, there is little tendency for recurrence. That said, however, there is seldom any indication to perform the procedure, particularly as it may be associated with significant complication rates.

Traumatic dislocation of the hip

Traumatic hip dislocation in children is rare. As it differs in many respects from the same disorder in adults, experience of the adult condition cannot be extrapolated to help us deal with children. In common with any traumatic condition in childhood, boys predominate, the male:female ratio being around 2:1 (Glass & Powell 1961, Funk 1962). Around two-thirds of all dislocations in childhood are the result of trivial injuries (Glass & Powell 1961), the younger the child the less the force required to produce dislocation. Offierski (1981), for example, found that 50% of children below the age of 10 dislocated as a result of minor trauma whereas all children above that age had been subjected to a moderate or severe degree of trauma.

The vast majority of cases dislocate posteriorly. The child thus presents with a history of injury, inability to walk, a flexed adducted hip and a shortened limb. The radiographic diagnosis is straightforward (Fig. 11.3). As in adults, if the diagnosis is missed it is usually because other injuries are present, particularly a fracture of the ipsilateral femur or a severe head injury. Whereas associated fractures, particularly of the acetabulum are present in around 75% of adults with hip dislocations, they are much less common in children, the reported incidence varying from none (Funk 1962, Offierski 1981) to 18% (Pennsylvania Orthopaedic Society 1968).

Most cases can be managed by closed methods, reduction being most easily obtained in younger children where the dislocating force has been trivial. It is worth emphasizing that the attempted reduction should be performed with some gentleness as excessive force may cause displacement of the upper femoral epiphysis from the neck (Fiddian & Grace 1983). Presuming the postreduction radiograph to be satisfactory, immobilization in a hip spica for around 6 weeks followed by a return to complete weightbearing on removal of the cast is sufficient treatment.

Only a small number require open reduction, usually those in whom the dislocating trauma has been severe or when the diagnosis has been delayed. If there is an ipsilateral fracture of the femur, then open reduction will be required because of the lack of control over the proximal fragment. Similarly, open reduction is indicated if, after an attempted closed reduction, the hip does not appear perfectly congruous. A posterior approach is best as the most common cause for post

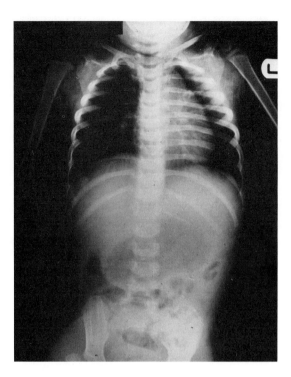

Fig. 11.3 A young child found in the back seat of a car which had been involved in an accident. Both her parents in the front seat were killed. Hip dislocation was not suspected clinically!

reduction incongruity is an inverted limbus which can best be visualized from the back (Offierski 1981). Once everted, reduction is usually possible. Whichever method of treatment is required, it should be undertaken with the least possible delay as there is no doubt that, the longer the hip is left dislocated, the worse will be the result.

The late diagnosed case presents problems of its own. If the hip has been out for some considerable time it may be that disuse osteoporosis will make attempted closed reduction hazardous. In that case, skeletal traction via a distal femoral pin can be used as an alternative method of reduction (Bonnel & Webster 1980).

Complications

The early complications include noncongruent reduction due to soft tissue interposition as discussed above and nerve palsies whilst, amongst the later complications avascular necrosis, recurrent dislocation and traumatic degenerative disease predominate.

Nerve palsy

Nerve palsies are uncommon. Wilchinsky and Pappas (1985) estimated that around 3% of dislocations were complicated by a sciatic nerve palsy. Pearson and Mann

(1973) reported 5 cases, all of which had some return of function although in only one was this complete. There have been isolated reports of other nerves being similarly damaged including the peroneal (Barquet 1979) and superior gluteal (Wilchinsky & Pappas 1985).

Avascular necrosis

Avascular necrosis will succeed hip dislocation in around 10% of cases (Pennsylvania Orthopaedic Society 1968) and is usually obvious within one year of injury. It is commonest in older children and indeed is almost unknown below the age of six (Hammelbo 1976). This, of course, may well be a reflection of the more severe trauma required to produce dislocation in the older age group. On the other hand, the direction of dislocation, the period of immobilization or of restriction of weightbearing seem not to have any effect upon the likelihood of its developing (Barquet 1982).

Recurrent dislocation

Age seems to be the only factor which predisposes to recurrence. Whilst most dislocations occur in late childhood or adolescence, recurrences are more often found in younger children (Barquet 1980). In the event of this happening, an arthrogram should be performed. If no abnormality can be demonstrated then it must be presumed that the capsule has merely been stretched and a further period of immobilization in a hip spica is required. If, however, sacculation or a tear is demonstrated then repair, usually via a posterior approach is carried out and a successful result can be anticipated.

Longterm results

The majority of children who sustain a traumatic dislocation of the hip will have good result both clinically and radiographically. Around one–third, however, will not. The most comprehensive series was published by the Pennsylvania Orthopaedic Society (1968) who followed up 44 children to skeletal maturity. Sixteen were found to have radiological abnormalities at final review. They concluded that the most important factor vis-á-vis the final result was the severity of the initial trauma: the more severe the trauma the more the risk of a poor result. Poor results are therefore more likely in older children.

Recurrent dislocation of the hip

Although recurrent dislocation of the hip may occur in otherwise normal children, it is more usually found secondary to some underlying local or general abnormality. Amongst the former can be counted trauma, dysplasia and sepsis whilst the latter includes paralytic disorders and generalized ligamentous laxity.

Voluntary habitual dislocation of the hip in otherwise normal children is a rare occurrence. It has usually been reported in girls who can produce a clicking hip by flexing, adducting and internally rotating the joint. Pain is not a prominent feature. Differentiation from the more common 'snapping' hip should be possible by determining the position that produces the click. Whilst the bony architecture looks normal on conventional radiographs, CT scans have been used to show a defect in the posterior acetabular wall at the site of dislocation (Goldberg & Rousso 1984). Similar defects have been found at operation (Haddad & Drez 1974). The outlook for spontaneous resolution is good and most children seem gradually to give up the habit (Goldberg & Rousso 1984, Broudy & Scott 1975, Petterson *et al.* 1980). As with recurrent dislocation of the shoulder it is best looked upon as a form of manipulative behaviour and appropriate counselling should be offered.

Ligamentous laxity is a feature of several disorders including Down syndrome in which recurrent dislocation may affect as many as 1 in 20 children (Bennet *et al.* 1982). This usually first happens during the period of greatest ligamentous laxity, that is between the ages of 2 and 10 (Fig. 11.4). The dislocation, which occurs without there being a history of trauma, at first reduces spontaneously, but with increasing age this outcome becomes less likely, such that, by late childhood subluxation proceeding to chronic dislocation in adult life is the rule. Capsular plication, combined with femoral osteotomy if excessive anteversion is present, seems the most effective mode of treatment.

The Ehlers Danlos syndrome perhaps springs most readily to mind as a condition

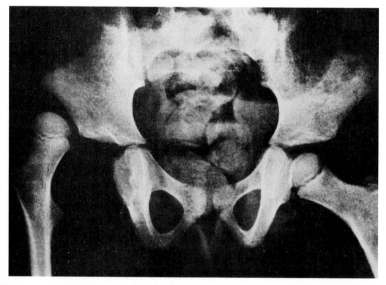

Fig. 11.4 Spontaneous dislocation of the hip in a six-yearold girl with Down syndrome. There was no history of trauma. The iliac bones are broad and the acetabular roof is horizontal, both characteristically found in Down syndrome.

associated with ligamentous laxity. Surprisingly, however, although the frequency of joint dislocation can be related to the degree of hypermobility in any particular patient, the hip is rarely affected (Beighton & Horan 1969).

Juvenile rheumatoid arthritis

Juvenile rheumatoid arthritis (JRA) affects around 1 in 1000 children under the age of 16 in the United Kingdom (Ansell & Swann 1983). Only a minority, however, will go on to develop chronic joint problems and indeed, 75% can be expected to make a full recovery (Schaller 1984). The differing patterns of behaviour of the various subtypes of the disease has led to a classification based on the presence or absence of systemic symptoms, the age and sex of the child at the time of its onset, the number of joints affected and the presence or absence of an IGM rheumatoid factor. All of these have some prognostic significance. For example, of those young children who develop the disease and have systemic symptoms, around half will develop a severe, and one in ten, a destructive arthritis (Ansell & Swann 1983). Similarly older girls who develop a polyarthritis and are seropositive have a poor prognosis as, in this group, the disease follows a course akin to rheumatoid arthritis in the adult. This contrasts with the excellent outlook for the younger child who develops pauciarticular disease.

The inflammatory changes of rheumatoid disease within the affected joint lead to pain, spasm and the development of periarticular contractures. As movement is lost subluxation, secondary to spasm in the psoas and the adductors, develops whilst the associated hyperaemia results in osteoporosis, overgrowth and eventually premature closure of the proximal femoral growth plate. These changes are evident radiologically as may be the features associated with adult disease namely cartilage loss, protrusio and ultimately degenerative changes (Fig. 11.5).

Surgery has little, if any, place in the early stages of the disease. If systemic symptoms predominate, bed rest, usually combined with skin traction and anti-inflammatory drugs is required. As a first line drug aspirin is usually effective but, if this does not control the systemic symptoms, steroids may need to be used. As the acute symptoms subside and the joint becomes more comfortable, mobilization, initially in the hydrotherapy pool, can be started. This is followed by a gradual progression to walking under the supervision of a physiotherapist once an adequate range of motion has been obtained. With such a regime many children settle down and the disease resolves. In others, however, it does not, becoming chronic, perhaps resulting in progressive joint destruction. Such children may benefit from surgery. Then, although hip joint involvement may appear to be the greatest barrier to the child's continued mobility, the symptoms arising from the hip cannot be considered in isolation. As the disease may be widespread, the degree of involvement elsewhere will certainly have an influence on surgical decisions with regard to their hip. For example, upper limb disease may mean that wallking aids could not be used postoperatively. Similarly, improved postoperative function of the hip may

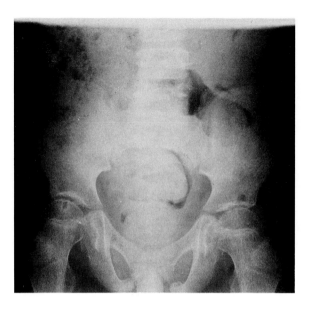

Fig. 11.5 The pelvic radiograph of a 7-year-old boy with polyarticular juvenile rheumatoid arthritis. Osteoporosis, loss of cartilage space, cyst formation and subluxation are all present.

exacerbate problems in other joints of the lower limbs. An attempt must be made to anticipate these problems.

As muscle spasm and contractures are the prime causes of deformity at the hip, their correction by soft tissue release is indicated in those children in whom medical therapy has failed. Such procedures should be undertaken before the joint is irreversibly damaged. Open adductor tenotomy and psoas release followed by splinting in a plaster shell in a position of extension and abduction is then the operation of choice. Once the postoperative discomfort has settled down, physiotherapy in the hydrotherapy pool can be started, returning to the plaster shell between sessions. It is acknowledged that the benefits of this operation are likely to be temporary. Although it will not alter the natural history of progression it is nevertheless a worthwhile procedure. Pain will be relieved and this will result in an improved range of motion. Particularly in the younger child, time will be gained to allow for further skeletal maturation before definitive operation is undertaken.

The effectiveness of synovectomy would appear to be comparable to that of soft tissue release. Results from centres with experience of this procedure suggest that, whilst temporary pain relief can be expected, it makes little difference to the progression of the disease. Nor does it result in an increased range of motion although some improvement in the hip position can be obtained (Jacobsen *et al.* 1985, Albright *et al.* 1975). In view of this there would appear to be little advantage in performing synovectomy rather than the simpler soft tissue release as both can be looked upon as holding procedures postponing the need for total hip replacement until skeletal maturity has been reached.

Other surgical procedures have little to offer. Osteoporosis make the fixation of osteotomies uncertain and as a result means that postoperative immobilization must be used. This increases the risk of stiffness developing. Likewise arthrodesis has no place in a bilateral condition in which every effort should be made to preserve whatever movement is present.

If, in spite of soft tissue release, degenerative joint disease develops and is interfering with function to an extent that the use of a wheelchair seems necessary then total hip replacement should be considered. Potential problems abound. Temperomandibular and cervical spine involvement may make anaesthesia difficult and intubation impossible (Mogensen *et al.* 1983, Bisla *et al.* 1976). The quality of the bone on both sides of the joint is likely to be poor. As a result of stunted growth the acetabulum may be underdeveloped. On the femoral side valgus and anteversion of the neck are often found (Bisla *et al.* 1976). This abnormal anatomy may necessitate the use of a custom built prosthesis. The widest possible surgical exposure should be obtained, this being best achieved by removal of the greater trochanter as in the Charnley approach. Because of extreme osteoporosis, reaming should be performed with extreme care as perforation of the cortex, particulary in the femoral shaft, is a real danger. Blood loss can be expected to be large, in one series averaging 78% of the blood volume (Roach & Paradies 1978). In spite of all these difficulties the results can be gratifying and when performed in units with special experience of the problem, remarkably good (Ansell & Swann 1983, Bisla *et al.* 1976, Mogensen *et al.* 1983, Morris *et al.* 1978). The vast majority of their patients obtained relief of pain and increased motion, as indicated by a reduction in their requirements for walking aids, their ultimate mobility only being limited by the extent of the disease in other lower limb joints. Loosening and progressive protrusio certainly occur but neither has proved to be as common as might be expected. Only time will tell whether the patients will outlive their prostheses and this will no doubt depend upon their level of activity.

Haemophilia

Haemophilia is a haemorrhagic disorder caused by a deficiency of one of the factors necessary for clotting to take place, Factor VIII in the case of haemophilia A and Factor IX in haemophilia B (Christmas disease). Both are inherited in a sex linked mode and are transmitted from a heterozygous carrier mother to her affected son.

The clinical manifestations of the disease depend upon the amount of factor present, this usually being expressed as a percentage of normal. Thus, when it is say 50%, the person is usually asymptomatic whereas, at levels of less than 1% symptoms are correspondingly more likely to be severe and to include spontaneous haemarthroses and intramuscular bleeds. It is such patients, within the severely affected category, who are likely to require orthopaedic aid.

The hip is seldom involved. In a study of 366 acute haemarthroses in 113 patients, Duthie *et al.* (1972) found the hip to be affected in only 5 (157 involved the knee, 109 the elbow and 73 the ankle). When it is, the symptoms are those of an acute haemarthrosis in any joint namely pain, associated with limitation of movement, and the adoption of a flexed posture. Pain in the region of the hip can also arise as a result of iliac haematoma but, the presence of a swelling in the iliac fossa combined with the signs of a femoral nerve palsy should allow the clinical distinction to be made. If doubt exists ultrasound will demonstrate the presence or otherwise of a haematoma.

The principles of treatment of an acute haemarthrosis are the same whichever joint is affected, these being rest, factor replacement and rehabilitation. In the case of the hip rest is best achieved by supporting the lower limb on the affected side on pillows to maintain the joint in the position of maximum comfort. This is accompanied by factor replacement sufficient to raise the factor level to between 30% to 50% of normal.

Once the acute discomfort has subsided, but still under factor cover, the child is successively mobilized in bed, in the hydrotherapy pool, finally proceeding to graduated weightbearing.

As the hip is rarely affected secondary changes are correspondingly rare but repeated haemarthrosis can be expected to produce avasucular necrosis and ultimately degenerative joint disease (Fig. 11.6). Whilst there is no doubt that such joint disease is still a serious cause of disability in the haemophiliac population, the outlook has been transformed by home therapy programmes in which factor is given either at the first sign of a bleed or alternatively on a twice weekly prophylactic basis. Using these regimes, destructive joint disease has become much less common.

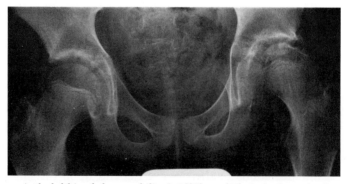

Fig. 11.6 Changes in the left hip of a haemophiliac (<1%) boy of 12 who had sustained repeated 'minor' bleeds into the joint.

Sickle cell disease

Sickle cell disease is a severe haemolytic anaemia found usually, but not exclusively, in negroes. The globin part of the haemoglobin molecule which is genetically determined, is normally characterized as HbA (adult haemoglobin). Minor changes in the amino acid sequence produce HbS (sickle cell haemoglobin). This has functional differences from normal adult haemoglobin in that, under conditions of reduced oxygen tension, it tends to come out of solution and crystallize. If the proportion of such abnormal haemoglobin is low, as in heterozygotes (HbAS, sickle cell trait) then the clinical effect is mild but, when an individual is homozygous (HbSS) practically all of the haemoglobin is abnormal and the clinical effects severe. Other abnormal haemoglobin may combine with HbS to produce double heterozygotes as in Hb thal, which may affect whites, HbSC and HbSF. These individuals have sickle cell disease albeit usually of a milder variety than the homozygous type. The gene of the abnormal haemoglobin is common in Africans or wherever the population is of African descent. For example 10.9% of Jamaicans have been found to have an HbSS electrophoretic pattern (Golding *et al.* 1959).

Crystallization of the abnormal haemoglobin results in venous stasis, thrombosis and infarction. Any system or organ may be affected. In the skeleton the effects can be due to either thrombosis or the associated anaemia. Chronic anaemia produces stunting of growth in childhood whilst secondary marrow hyperplasia causes osteoporosis and cortical thinning, this being particularly evident in the vertebrae and the skull. Thrombosis and infarction occur most commonly in the femoral head, such changes affecting up to 12% of the sickle cell population (Chung 1981, Iwegbu & Fleming 1985). Three different patterns of femoral head involvement have been described. Partial head involvement resembling Perthes disease is most common in younger children whereas in the older age group the whole head may be involved producing gross destruction and eventually severe deformity (Chung & Ralston 1969). In the third type a localized infarct followed by a subchondral fracture produces the appearance of osteochondritis dissecans (Washington & Root 1985). In general, the severity of symptoms is related to the extent of head involvement. Thus whilst Perthes-like changes produce only mild to moderate pain, those with osteochondritis dissecans or whole head involvement are likely to suffer severe discomfort.

The diagnosis usually presents little problem particularly if it is remembered that a diagnosis of Perthes disease should be accepted in a negro patient only if the electrophoretic pattern is known to be normal.

The treatment and prognosis too depend upon the pattern of the disease. In the Perthes type prolonged partial weightbearing has been shown to produce good results, even when growth is almost complete (Washington & Root 1985). If subluxation occurs, varus osteotomy as in Perthes disease is probably indicated. In the osteochondritic type the same procedure can be used to shift the weightbearing area within the femoral head as spontaneous healing of such a defect is most unlikely. Total head involvement represents end stage disease and consequently only salvage procedures are possible (Fig. 11.7).

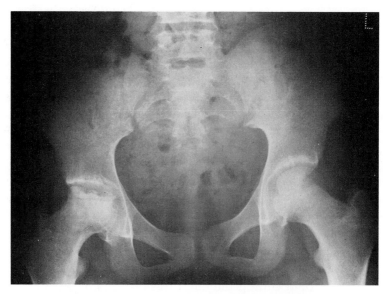

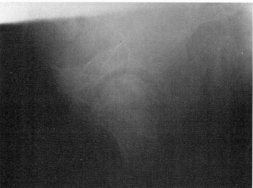

Fig. 11.7 The hip radiographs of a 15-year-old Nigerian girl with avascular necrosis of the right femoral head. Her electrophoretic pattern was HbSS.

Leukaemia

The commonest of childhood malignancies, leukaemia is a primary disorder of bone marrow in which the marrow elements are replaced by immature or undifferentiated blast cells. Its importance from an orthopaedic point of view stems from the fact that, in the vast majority of cases, bone involvement is present at some stage of the disease. Indeed, in around 20% bone pain, usually in the lower limb, is one of the presenting features (Rogalsky *et al.* 1986). As the peak incidence of the disease is between the ages of 2 and 5 years, such a symptom, especially if combined with refusal to weightbear, may initially suggest one of the more common orthopaedic complaints such as transient synovitis. This merely emphasizes the need for a general, as well as local examination in any limb disorder as lymphadenopathy, clinical anaemia and splenomegaly are likely to be present.

The radiographic features of leukaemia are not specific enough to make a confident diagnosis. A combination of periosteal elevation, osteoporosis and cystic areas produces a moth-eaten appearance (Fig. 11.8). A skeletal survey usually reveals the presence of other similar lesions elsewhere in the body. The diagnosis can usually be made on a blood sample with anaemia being present in 80% and thrombocytopenia in a similar proportion (Jones *et al.* 1976). Marrow examination is confirmatory.

Prior to the introduction of chemotherapy practically all affected children were dead within 6 months, whereas since, some 90% obtain a remission. Lanzkowsky (1983) estimated that 50% of such children can be expected to survive 5 years and perhaps half of those might ultimately prove to be cured. Chemotherapeutic agents themselves may cause musculoskeletal problems. Bone pain and pathological fractures, occasionally refractory to union, are particularly associated with the use of methotrexate (Ragab *et al.* 1970).

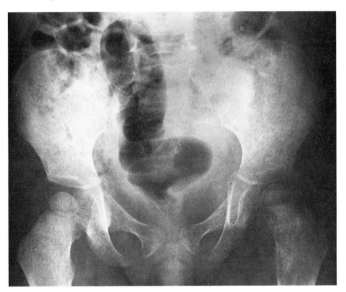

Fig. 11.8 The pelvic radiograph of a 6-year-old girl referred as transient synovitis causing a limp on the left side. She resented her left leg being handled and there was concentric reduction of the range of motion of the left hip. The proximal left femur shows the moth-eaten appearance of leukaemic infiltrate.

Idiopathic chondrolysis

Whilst chondrolysis has long been known to develop in a proportion of children affected by slipping of the capital femoral epiphysis, trauma, burns or prolonged immobilization, it was only in 1971 that Jones described its occurrence in otherwise normal children, usually black adolescent females, in the absence of any of these predisposing factors.

Its aetiology is unknown although an auto-immune cause has been suggested on the basis of elevated immunoglobulin and complement levels (Mankin *et al.* 1975). There is no evidence that infection plays a part. The histopathological changes are unhelpful. Synovial thickening, associated with nonspecific synovitis and fibrillation of the articular cartilage, particularly in the femoral side of the joint, have been consistently described but give little clue to the causation of the condition. (Duncan *et al.* 1979).

Clinically the disease is of insidious onset with pain in the hip and a limp being the earliest symptoms. The limb is characteristically held in flexion, adduction and internal rotation and a severe fixed flexion deformity may develop (Jones 1971). Motion is concentrically reduced, this becoming gradually more severe until the joint is almost ankylosed. Blood tests including the ESR are normal. Radiographs show osteoporosis followed by a decrease in the cartilage space to 1 mm to 2 mm (normal 3 mm to 5 mm). Eventually osteoarthritic changes develop (*see* Fig. 8.14).

As this is an uncommon disease, the temptation to explore the joint in the early stages to exclude other, more common pathologies such as infection, is almost irresistable. Once the diagnosis has been confirmed, bedrest combined with the use of Hamilton–Russel traction is advisable in the acute stage. Nonweightbearing exercises can be given. Continuous passive motion is certainly worth trying although the effectiveness of this mode of treatment is uncertain. Aspirin, to therapeutic levels, should be given on an empirical basis.

Once the acute stage has settled down then graduated weightbearing, initially with crutches, should be started, returning to skin traction when in bed. If, in spite of these measures, deformity persists or marked joint stiffness remains, then corrective soft tissue release would seem advisable as the aim at this stage is to keep the hip in a functional position. Irrespective of how they are treated, most affected hips become ankylosed although this may take up to 18 months. A few show some recovery (Duncan 1970) so that definitive procedures such as arthrodesis or resurfacing should not be performed prematurely and certainly not within 2 years of the onset of the disease.

Epiphyseal dysplasias

The epiphyseal dysplasias are a heterogenous group of disorders characterized by defective epiphyseal growth and ossification. Although their exact prevelance is unknown, all are uncommon (Wynne-Davies & Hall 1982). Whilst any epiphysis may be involved, the proximal femur is often the most severely so and indeed may be the only one affected. Hip incongruity and degenerative joint disease result. Although no specific treatment is available, an exact diagnosis is desirable as only then can an accurate prognosis be given, genetic advice offered and ineffective treatment avoided.

The two most common types to affect the hip are multiple epiphyseal dysplasia (MED) and spondyloepiphyseal dysplasia (SED). In the former the ossific nucleus of the proximal femoral epiphysis is late in appearing and, when it does, has a stippled appearance. With growth it becomes irregular and eventually flattened and deformed. Secondary deformity of the acetabulum results.

From a clinical point of view the severity of the symptoms reflect the severity of the radiographic changes. When these changes are mild there may be no discomfort referable to the hip until adolescence or early adult life but, as is more common, when the changes are extensive, hip pain and stiffness, usually accompanied by a waddling gait, are evident in childhood. Degenerative joint disease follows by the third or fourth decade (Spranger 1976).

In spondyloepiphyseal dysplasia the spinal changes are clinically more immediately obvious as platyspondyly produces short trunk dwarfism. In this type the ossific nucleus is again late in appearing. Once again the femoral head becomes flattened and mishapen and this, combined with often severe coxa vara and bowing of the proximal femur contribute to futher loss of stature. In the later onset type, the changes are less severe and coxa vara is not present. Children with this type tend to become symptomatic between the ages of 5 and 10 and by 40 years of age osteoarthritis is established. Differentiating this less severe type from multiple epiphyseal dysplasia may be difficult as the spinal changes are minimal and the children's stature may be within the normal range.

From a clinical viewpoint, the most important diagnostic conundrum is that between one of the epiphyseal dysplasias and bilateral Perthes disease. Radiographs of the spine and wrists, in addition to those of the pelvis, may reveal more generalized changes inconsistent with Perthes disease. The local hip changes may be of help. Whereas in epiphyseal dysplasia the two sides tend to have symmetrical changes, the opposite is true in Perthes disease where they tend to be asymmetrical each hip being at a different stage of the disease. Also, whilst metaphyseal changes are the rule in Perthes disease they are unusual in the dysplasias (Crossan *et al.* 1983).

There is no specific treatment for a hip affected by one of these disorders. Simple remedies such as crutch walking or hydrotherapy may tide the patient over the more acute periods. Whilst the effects of femoral osteotomies have not been evaluated it would appear to be an appropriate procedure when coxa vara is present. That said, however, there is nothing that we can offer to reverse the progression of the disease and total joint replacement at an early age remains the likeliest outcome.

Synovial osteochondromatosis

This is an unusual condition of unknown aetiology which seldom affects children. Although the knee is most commonly involved, any diarthrodial joint may be affected. Pathologically the characteristic feature is metaplasia of the synovium. This results in the production of osteocartilagenous lesions which are extruded into the joint as loose bodies. It is, however, a self limiting condition for eventually the synovium ceases to produce such lesions and indeed, resorption of previously formed loose bodies may even occur (Pelker *et al.* 1983, McIvor & King 1962). Only a small number of cases affecting the hip have been described. Muscular atrophy, crepitation, catching, giving way, pain and stiffness or indeed any combination of these may be found. That said, it is unlikely that the diagnosis will even be suspected on clinical grounds. In the early stages of the disease the X-ray will be of little help. Osteoporosis and an increase in the normal joint space may be present (Milgram & Pease 1980). If the diagnosis is considered arthrography is indicated. More often, the diagnosis is not made until radio-opaque loose bodies are evident or alternatively, at exploratory arthrotomy.

Treatment consists of removal of the abnormal synovium and loose bodies. Using a Smith–Peterson approach, the hip capsule is opened and the femoral head dislocated. Only a very incomplete synovectomy can be performed without doing so. All the loose bodies are removed and the joint washed out. Postoperatively a one-and-a-half hip spica for 6 weeks followed by physiotherapy, initially in the hydrotherapy pool, is indicated.

Fibrous dysplasia

Fibrous dysplasia is an uncommon condition of unknown aetiology in which fibro-osseous tissue proliferates within bone destroying its normal structure. There are two forms the more common monostotic, and polyostotic. In the former only one bone, often the femur,is affected whereas, in the latter, several are involved, sometimes all within one limb, occasionally only on one side of the body but more usually throughout the skeleton. The polyostotic variety, which tends to cause more severe deformities, may be associated with skin pigmentation and precocious puberty (Albright syndrome). Such findings are exceedingly rare in the monostotic type (Nakashima et al. 1984).

Both types have a predilection for the proximal femur. When bone is replaced, structural stability is lost and deformity results. Whereas in the monostotic variety the lesion tends to be confined to the femoral neck, in the polyostotic it typically extends into the shaft resulting in bowing and a shepherd's crook deformity. A fracture through such a deformed area or the deformity itself are the usual presenting features.

The radiographic changes may demonstrate a very variable degree of involvement. The lesions are characteristically cystic and multilobulated with thinning of the overlying cortex (Fig. 11.9). In the polyostotic variety the geography of the lesions normally makes the diagnosis straightforward, whereas, if monostotic it may be less clear cut and enchondroma, aneurysmal bone cyst, eosinophilic granuloma, unicameral bone cyst and nonosteogenic fibroma may need to be excluded by biopsy. If structural stability is threatened then surgery is indicated. If the femur is undeformed, curettage and packing the resultant cavity with bone graft may be all that is required. In general, a good result can be anticipated, particularly in the monostotic variety (Nakashima et al. 1984). Prophylactic fixation is indicated if the lesion is large. In the polyostotic variety, as coxa vara often coexists, the bone grafting procedure should be combined with valgus osteotomy.

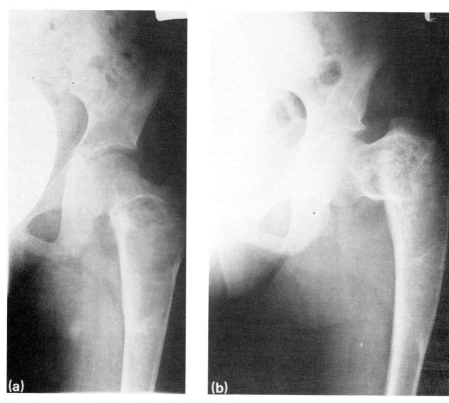

Fig. 11.9 (a) Polystotic fibrous dysplasia involving both the femoral neck and proximal shaft. (b) Progressive coxa vara is the result.

The results of such surgery are less predictable and repeated osteotomies may be required (Funk & Wells 1973).

Tumours and cysts

Most benign and malignant tumours of childhood can affect the hip joint region. That said, however, the site is not one of special predilection and the behaviour of tumours in this region is no different to that elsewhere. Their management though, is dictated by the particular anatomy of the hip and this may certainly cause problems.

The early symptoms of a neoplasm, whether benign or malignant, may mimic those of more common hip disorders leading to a delay in diagnosis. Unlike other locations, the appearance or palpation of a lump is not the usual presenting complaint, the majority being brought to attention by the presence of pain, a pathological fracture or, in the case of benign lesions, as an incidental finding on a radiograph taken for some other reason.

The anatomy of the hip joint affects the surgical management in two ways. Biopsy must be carefully planned so as not to produce excessive weakening of the femur, thus minimising the risk of producing a pathological fracture. Access may be difficult. A lesion in the head can usually be reached via a window in the anterior aspect of the neck whereas, if the lesion lies within the neck then an opening in the cortex below the greater trochanter, combined with the use of X-ray control allows access. If, at the time of biopsy the growth appears benign, then definitive curettage can be performed. Even with such conservative surgery, stability may be jeopardized to an extent that internal fixation appears advisable.

Benign tumours

Bone cysts

Simple bone cysts are usually found in late childhood, that is between the ages of 5 and 10 and are most often located in either the proximal femur or humerus. Exactly how common they are is unknown as it is likely that many remain asymptomatic and consequently undiagnosed before disappearing at skeletal maturity. They seldom give rise to pain, around two-thirds being diagnosed as a consequence of a pathological fracture, most of the remainder coming to light as a result of serendipity. The age, location, radiological features and the presence of fluid on aspiration determines the diagnosis. If there is any doubt, open biopsy is indicated. When they are asymptomatic and there is no risk to the mechanical integrity of the skeleton, observation at regular intervals is sufficient. Around the hip, however, this is often not the case as the risk of a fracture or growth disturbance is often very real.

Until recently, surgery, usually in the form of curettage and bone grafting, was the accepted method of treatment. The results were mixed with an overall recurrence rate of 15–40%. The outcome of such surgery in young children with active cysts was even worse with the recurrence rate in this subgroup reaching 88% (Openheim & Galleno 1984). Whilst better results can be obtained with more radical surgery such as subtotal diaphysectomy (Feller et al. 1982) such methods are clearly not applicable in the region of the proximal femur.

Since Scaglietti et al. (1979) introduced the technique of steroid injections this method of treatment has gained widespread acceptance. It is best performed under general anaesthesia. Two number 18 spinal needles with the stylets in situ are introduced into the cyst. The stylets are removed once correct positioning of the needles has been confirmed radiographically and the straw coloured fluid within the cyst allowed to escape. Saline is then instilled via one needle and allowed to drain from the other until the recovered fluid is clear. One needle is then removed and methylprednisolone acetate is introduced via the remaining one. The amount instilled does not appear to be vital. Campanna et al. (1982) recommend between 80 mg and 200 mg depending upon the size of the cyst. The needle is then removed.

If there seems to be a risk of a pathological fracture then crutch walking is advisable until such time as healing is underway. When pain in the cyst has been a feature, it is often dramatically relieved and indeed may have disappeared on recovery from the anaesthetic. Radiographic follow up is essential (Fig. 11.10). A satisfactory response is indicated by the cessation of expansion of the cyst and thickening of the surrounding cortex. The central radiolucent defect becomes progressively radio-opaque initially taking on a frosted glass appearance and eventually filling in completely. If an inadequate response is obtained then the injection can be repeated at 2 to 3 monthly intervals.

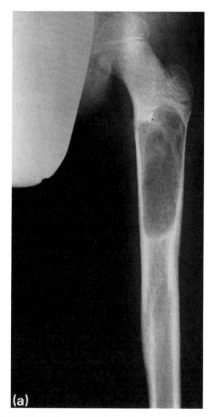
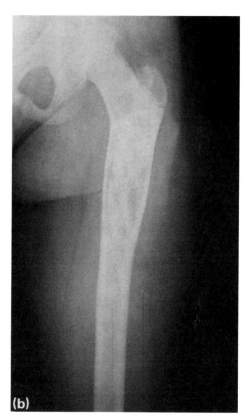

Fig. 11.10 A 14-year-old boy who presented complaining of pain in the thigh and a limp. (a) A simple bone cyst was present. This was treated by saline washout and instilling 120 mg methyl prednisolone acetate. Immediate pain relief was obtained. (b) Six months later satisfactory infilling of the cyst is evident.

The results of this simple technique are gratifying and a 75–95% success rate can be anticipated (Campanna *et al.* 1982, Malawar *et al.* 1985, Oppenheim & Galleno 1984, Smith *et al.* 1985), although in each series, a proportion of patients required repeated injection before a successful outcome was obtained. Whilst there was a higher rate of failure to respond below the age of 5, activity of the cyst or previous surgery seemed to have no bearing on the final result. In summary, the injection technique achieves superior results to those obtained by surgery, and this, combined with a much lower morbidity rate, means that surgery is no longer the treatment of choice. Future refinement of the more conservative technique will certainly occur. It is, for example, uncertain what effect the steroid has on the cyst as good results have been obtained by merely washing out the cyst and by the use of multiple puncture techniques (Chigura *et al.* 1983).

Osteoid osteoma

Osteoid osteoma is an uncommon benign tumour of bone affecting mainly adolescents and young adults, the peak incidence being in the second decade. Males are affected twice as commonly as females. Around 5% occur in the femoral neck (Johnson 1955) usually on the medial border of the calcar above the lesser trochanter or in the intertrochanteric line. From a pathological point of view it is an unusual lesion in that it has a very limited growth potential, the nucleus seldom reaching a diameter of more than 1 cm. Additionally, the area of sclerosis surrounding the central vascular nucleus may be many times greater in diameter than the nucleus itself. As it is seldom found after the age of 30, it would seem likely that is runs a self-limiting course (Moberg 1951, Golding 1954). Healing occurs by calcification of the nucleus but the time this might take has been estimated at anything betwen 2 and 24 years (Enneking 1983).

Clinically pain is the cardinal feature. Unrelated to activity, it is at first intermittent but later becomes constant, increasing in severity and characteristically being most troublesome at night. In about half the cases, it is referred to the knee. The excellent analgesic effect of salicytates as opposed to that of other mild analgesics is usually considered to be of diagnostic significance (Sim *et al.* 1975). The clinical signs produced are subtle consisting of muscle wasting in the buttock and thigh and perhaps slight restriction of hip movement secondary to synovitis. Occasionally, if the tumour is located adjacent to the growth plate, a disturbance of growth producing a leg length discrepancy may be found (Norman & Dorfmann 1975). The nonspecific nature of the pain and the relative lack of physical findings may lead to a considerable delay in diagnosis (Jackson *et al.* 1977, Goldberg & Jacobs 1975). Often a year may elapse before the correct diagnosis is made and, in the interim period, hysteria is not uncommonly suspected. The delay may to some extent be accounted for by the fact that the onset of pain may predate the development of radiological changes. The characteristic X-ray appearance is of a central radiolucent nucleus surrounded by an area of sclerosis (Fig. 11.11). Regional osteoporosis may also be present (Spence & Lloyd-Roberts 1961). The classical changes are, however, only found in around two-thirds of patients (Omojola *et al.* 1981, Swee *et al.* 1979).

If the clinical suspicion exists, then even in the absence of radiographic changes, further investigations, including tomography and radioisotope bone scanning, should be undertaken. Tomograms will often demonstrate a nucleus not visible on plain films. A positive bone scan is characterized by a localized area of increased uptake on both the 5 minute blood pool film and 2 hour delayed film. The increased early uptake differentiates osteoid osteoma from a stress fracture, both of which have similar appearances in the delayed film. There is usually too a diffusely increased uptake around the hip reflecting the coexisting synovitis. Whilst a CT scan may demonstrate the nucleus it does not contribute to the surgical management and so is unnecessary.

In the presence of the classic radiographic changes the diagnosis is not too difficult as no other lesion will produce an area of surrounding sclerosis many

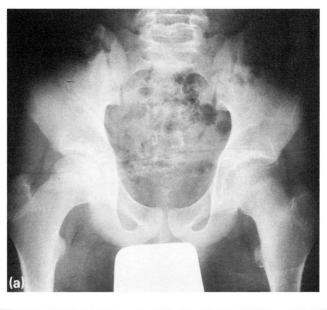

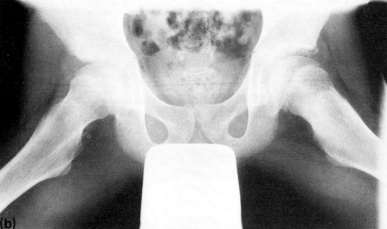

Fig. 11.11 (a) and (b) Radiographs of a 10-year-old girl who complained of pain in the left hip. There is an area of sclerosis in the neck.

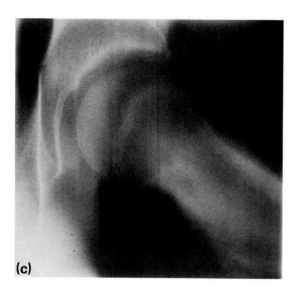

(c)

(c) Tomograms of the hip confirm the presence of a nidus.

times the size of the primary focus. Otherwise osteosarcoma, Ewings tumour, stress fractures and particularly a Brodie's abscess might all be considered.

Although there is a reflex action to suggest surgical excision, it is worth remembering that this is a self-limiting condition. If the symptoms are not too bad it is not unreasonable to suggest a period of salicylate analgesia and observation. The acute phase of the pain requiring analgesia normally settles within 36 months although the nucleus may not show signs of healing for several years (Enneking 1983). Often such a course is not possible and surgical treatment is the rule. As at operation the bone overlying the lesion is likely to be indistinguishable from the surrounding bone, the first problem is one of localization. Intraoperative radiographs are essential. An alternative is to use a radioactivity detector probe during the procedure, having first administered a dose of 99m TC in the immediate preoperative period (Colton & Hardy 1983, Kumar *et al.* 1984). Once the area of high activity is found the cortex is windowed and curettage is performed until the radioactivity count is the same in that region as in the backgound bone. Curettage, rather than *en bloc* excision is the preferred method of treatment in the hip region. Even after such a conservative procedure bone grafting and internal fixation may still be required. Whatever surgical procedure is used, the outlook is excellent and relief of symptoms is usually evident as soon as the patient recovers from anaesthesia.

Eosinophilic granuloma

Eosinophilic granulomata represent the localized, benign part of the spectrum of the disorder Histiocytosis-X. The generalized forms, namely Letterer–Siewe and Hand–Schüller–Christian disease have a less favourable prognosis. All are disorders of the lymphoreticular system, characterized by histiocytic and eosinophilic lymphocyte infiltrations of the affected tissues although their aetiology remains a matter for speculation. Most cases arise in the first three decades of life with a peak being found between the ages of 5 and 10. Around one-quarter will involve the pelvis or the femur (Fowler & Bobechko 1970). Localized pain is the usual presenting feature. The radiographic appearance is that of a well demarcated round or oval translucency, occasionally associated with periosteal reaction which may be lamellated giving an 'onion skin' appearance (this may also be a feature of Ewing tumour, osteosarcoma, osteomyelitis and secondary deposits, particularly neuroblastoma) (Fig. 11.12).

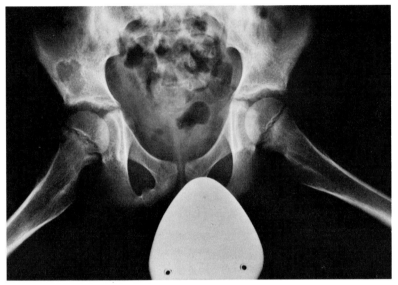

Fig. 11.12 An eosinophilic granuloma in a common location immediately above the acetabulum. The appearance is typical: a cystic lesion with well defined sharply demarcated borders.

Eosinophilic granulomata are benign lesions which tend to heal spontaneously (Sartoris & Parker 1984). Intervention is required only if the diagnosis is in doubt, in which case, biopsy should be performed, or if by reason of its position, a pathological fracture seems likely or if pain is a prominent feature. If biopsy is undertaken it seems reasonable to pack the cavity with bone chips although it has to be said that there is no evidence that this increases the incidence of healing (Enneking 1983). In future it may be that needle biopsy and instillation of methylprednisolone, as in the treatment of simple bone cysts, will prove to be the treatment of choice (Leeson *et al.* 1985, Cohen *et al.* 1980).

Aneurysmal bone cysts

These usually occur in adolescence or early adult life, characteristically arising in the metaphysis of a long bone or the pelvis. Their behaviour is variable ranging from that similar to a bone cyst to those with progression more like that of a sarcoma. Clinically they may produce a variable degree of local discomfort, a pelvic mass, a painful limp, limitation of hip motion or, on occasion, a pathological fracture. Radiographs show a cystic lesion contained within an intact, but very much thinned, margin of cortex (Fig. 11.13). Although in the older adolescent patient a giant cell tumour may have a similar radiographic appearance, there is usually little doubt about the diagnosis. Curettage and packing of the cavity with bone chips can be expected to lead to resolution in some 70% (Enneking 1983) although Cole (1986) has obtained satisfactory results by merely removing the soft tissue contents. In spite of such a satisfactory outcome being the rule, maintenance of stability may pose considerable problems.

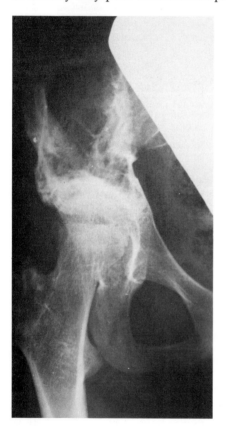

Fig. 11.13 An aneurysmal bone cyst in a 9-year-old girl who complained of pain on weightbearing and was locally tender over the ilium. The range of passive movements at the hip was normal.

Malignant tumours

Primary malignant bone tumours

Whilst osteosarcoma and chondrosarcoma may occur almost anywhere in the skeleton, the combination of one of these tumours arising in the hip region of a child is extremely rare. Chondrosarcoma usually presents in an older age group (Lichtenstein 1977). Lloyd-Roberts and Ratliff (1978) reported having seen only one case of osteosarcoma arising in the femoral neck and that was in a healing fracture in a child with osteogenesis imperfecta.

Ewing's tumour

Ewing's tumour is a primary malignant tumour of bone affecting mainly children and adolescents. The femur and innominate bones are commonly involved. Although usually presenting on account of localized pain or swelling, the associated systemic symptoms such as fever or weight loss may bring the tumour to light. So too may skeletal or pulmonary metastases which are present in 25% of children at the time of diagnosis.

Radiologically the appearance is of a destructive lesion, possibly with lines of periosteal new bone giving a lamellated 'onion skin' appearance. This may also be found in association with osteosarcomata and osteomyelitis. Differentiation from a neuroblastoma may be difficult, particularly as there may be histological similarities but estimation of urinary catecholamines usually allows the distinction to be made.

When the pelvis is affected the outlook is poor. The best method of treatment is still a matter of controversy. Generally, control of the primary tumour with radiotherapy, often preceded by chemotherapy is attempted. As yet, no one regime seems to give any particular advantage. If a satisfactory response is obtained, surgical excision may be feasible.

Secondary tumours

With the exception of spread from primary bone tumours, most secondary deposits in bone arise from that most common tumour of infancy, neuroblastoma. This takes origin from cells of the sympathetic nervous system and may therefore arise from any site where such nerve tissue is present. The embryonic nature of the tumour is manifest by its commonly occuring in early life, 50% appearing before the age of two and 75% before the age of 4. As 70% of children have skeletal metastases at the time of diagnosis these may well give rise to the presenting complaint. Radiologically such deposits appear either as single irregular destructive lesion, usually associated with an overlying periosteal reaction or as a diffuse infiltrate at the ends of long bones, in that case resembling leukaemic changes or perhaps a Ewing's sarcoma. Occasionally a pathological fracture may occur (Fig. 11.14). Because of the tissue of origin neuroblastomas usually secrete variable amounts of the metabolites of the catacholamines and these can be identified in the urine. Significantly raised levels of homovanillic acid (HVA) or vallinylmandelic acid (VMA) are found in over 90% of affected patients.

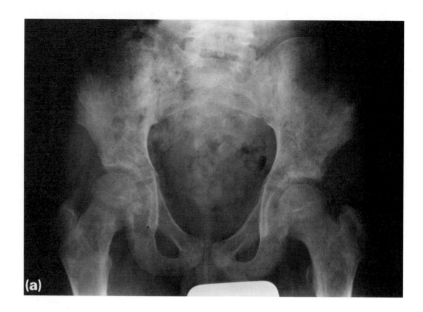

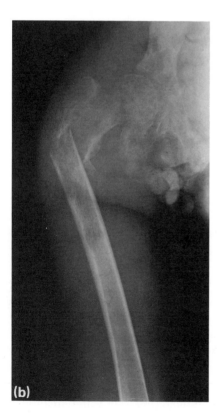

Fig. 11.14 (a) Widespread infiltrating bony deposits in neuroblastoma. Although the patient was bedbound, the lesion in the right femoral neck resulted in a fracture.
(b) This was treated conservatively in a Thomas splint at home and united satisfactorily shortly before the patient died.

Treatment consists of a variable combination of surgery, radiotherapy and chemotherapy depending upon the stage of the disease. Radiotherapy is particularly useful in relieving bone pain. Overall the prognosis is poor although, particularly below the age of one year, a small proportion undergo spontaneous regression. Otherwise the survival figures are inversely related to age, being around 74% below the age of one and 12% above the age of two years (Lanzkowsky 1983).

References

Torsional abnormalities

Coon V., Donald G., Houser C., Bleck E. E. (1975) Normal ranges of hip motion in infants between 3 months and 6 months of age. *Clinical Orthopedics and Related Research*, **110**, 256–60.

Dunlap K., Shands A. R., Hollister L. C., Gaul J. S. & Streit H. A. (1953) A new method of determination of torsion of the femur. *Journal of Bone and Joint Surgery*, **35A**, 289–311.

Dunn D. (1952) Anteversion of the neck of the femur. *Journal of Bone and Joint Surgery*, **34B**, 181–6.

Fabry G., McEwan G. D. & Shands A. R. (1973) Torsion of the femur. A follow up study in normal and abnormal conditions. *Journal of Bone and Joint Surgery*, **55A**, 1726–38.

Hubbard D. D. & Staheli I. T. (1972) The clinical treatment of femoral torsion with axial tomography. *Clinical Orthopedics and Related Research*, **86**, 16–20.

Kling T. F. & Hensinger R. N. (1983) Angular and torsion deformities of the two limbs in children. *Clinical Orthopedics and Related Research*, **186**, 136–42.

Luchini M. & Stevens D. B. (1983) The validity of torsional profile examination. *Journal of Pediatric Orthopedics*, **3**, 41–4.

McSweeney A. (1971) A study of femoral torsion in children. *Journal of Bone and Joint Surgery*, **53B**, 90–5.

Moulton A. & Upadhyay S. S. (1982) A direct method of treating femoral anteversion using ultrasound. *Journal of Bone and Joint Surgery*, **64B**, 469–72.

Phillips H. O., Greene W. B., Guilford W. B., Mittelstaedt C. A., Gaisie B., Vincent L. M. & Durell C. (1985) Measurement of femoral torsion: Comparison of standard roentogenographic techniques with ultrasound. *Journal of Pediatric Orthopedics*, **5**, 546–9.

Ryder C. T. & Crane L. (1953) Measuring femoral anteversion: The problems and a method. *Journal of Bone and Joint Surgery*, **35A**, 321–8.

Scrutton D. & Robson P. (1968) The gait of 50 normal children. *Physiotherapy*, **54**, 363–8.

Sharrard W. J. W. (1979) *Paediatric Orthopaedics and Fractures*, Blackwell Scientific Publications, Oxford.

Sommerville E. (1957) Persistent foetal alignment of the hip. *Journal of Bone and Joint Surgery*, **39B**, 106–113.

Staheli L. T. (1977) Torsional deformities *Pediatric Clinics of North America*, **24**, 799–811.

Staheli L. T., Lipper T. F. & Denotter P. (1977) Femoral anteversion and physical performance in adolescence and adult life. *Clinical Orthopedics and Related Research*, **129**, 213–16.

Traumatic dislocation of the hip

Barquet A. (1979) Traumatic hip dislocation in children. *Acta Orthopaedica Scandinavica*, **50**, 549–53.

Barquet A. (1980) Recurrent traumatic dislocation of the hip in children. *Journal of Trauma*, **20**, 1003–6.

Barquet A. (1982) Avascular necrosis following traumatic hip dislocation in children. *Acta Orthopaedica Scandinavica*, **53**, 809–13.

Broudy A. S. & Scott R. D. (1975) Voluntary posterior dislocation in children. A report of two cases. *Journal of Bone and Joint Surgery*, **57A**, 716–7.

Bunnell W. P. & Webster D. A. (1980) Late reduction of bilateral hip dislocation in a child. *Clinical Orthopedics and Related Research*, **147**, 160–3.

Fiddian N. J. & Grace D. L. (1983) Traumatic dislocation of the hip in adolescence with separation of the capital epiphysis: Two case reports. *Journal of Bone and Joint Surgery*, **65B**, 148–9.

Funk F. J. (1962) Traumatic dislocation of the hip in children. *Journal of Bone and Joint Surgery*, **44A**, 1135–45.

Glass A. & Powell H. D. W. (1961) Traumatic dislocation of the hip in children. *Journal of Bone and Joint Surgery,* **43B,** 29–37.

Hammelbo T. (1976) Traumatic dislocation of the hip in childhood. *Acta Orthopaedica Scandinavica,* **47,** 546–8.

Offierski C. M. (1981) Traumatic dislocation of the hip in children. *Journal of Bone and Joint Surgery,* **63B,** 194–7.

Pearson D. E. & Mann R. J. (1973) Traumatic dislocation of the hip in children. *Clinical Orthopedics and Related Research,* **92,** 189–94.

Pennsylvania Orthopaedic Society (1968) Traumatic dislocation of the hip joint in children. *Journal of Bone and Joint Surgery,* **50A,** 79–88.

Wilchinsky M. E. & Pappas A. M. (1985) Unusual complications in traumatic dislocation of the hip in children. *Journal of Pediatric Orthopedics,* **5,** 534–9.

Recurrent dislocation of the hip

Beighton P. & Horan F. (1969) Orthopaedic aspects of Ehlers–Danlos syndrome. *Journal of Bone and Joint Surgery,* **51B,** 444–53.

Bennet G. C., Rang M., Roye D. & Apron H. (1982) Dislocation of the hip in Trisomy 21. *Journal of Bone and Joint Surgery,* **64B,** 289–94.

Goldberg I. & Rousso I. (1984) Voluntary habitual dislocation of the hip: A case report with follow up by computerized tomography. *Journal of Bone and Joint Surgery,* **66A,** 1117–9.

Haddad R. J. & Drez D. (1974) Voluntary recurrent anterior dislocation of the hip. *Journal of Bone and Joint Surgery,* **56A,** 419–22.

Petterson H., Theander G. & Danielson L. (1980) Voluntary habitual dislocation of the hip in children. *Acta Radiologica Diagnostica,* **21,** 303–7.

Juvenile Rheumatoid Arthritis

Albright J. A., Albright J. P. & Ogden J. (1975) Synovectomy of the hip in juvenile rheumatoid arthritis. *Clinical Orthopedics and Related Research,* **106,** 48–55.

Ansell B. & Swann M. (1983) The management of chronic arthritis of children. *Journal of Bone and Joint Surgery,* **65B,** 536–43.

Bisla R. S., Inglis A. E. & Ranawat C. S. (1976) Joint replacement in patients under thirty. *Journal of Bone and Joint Surgery,* **58A,** 1098–104.

Jacobsen S., Levinson J. E. & Crawford A. H. (1985) Late results of synovectomy in juvenile rheumatoid arthritis. *Journal of Bone and Joint Surgery,* **67A,** 8–15.

Mogensen A., Brattstrom H., Ekedlund L. & Lidgren L. (1983) Total hip replacement in juvenile chronic arthritis. *Acta Orthopaedica Scandinavica,* **54,** 422–80.

Morris J., Ansell B. M. & Arden G. P. (1978) Total hip arthroplasty in juvenile chronic polyarthritis. *Journal of Bone and Joint Surgery,* **60B,** 288.

Roach J. W. & Paradies L. H. (1984) Total hip arthroplasty performed during adolescence. *Journal Pediatric Orthopedics,* **4,** 418–21.

Schaller J. G. (1984) Chronic arthritis in children. *Clinical Orthopedics and Related Research,* **182,** 79–89.

Haemophilia

Duthie R. B., Mathews J. M., Rizza C. R. & Steel W. (1972) *The Management of Musculoskeletal Problems in Haemophilia,* p. 30. Blackwell Scientific Publications, Oxford.

Sickle cell disease

Chung S. M. K. (1981) *Hip Disorders in Infants and Children,* pp. 299–309. Lea & Febiger, Philadelphia.

Chung S. M. K. & Ralston E. L. (1969) Necrosis of the femoral head associated with sickle cell anaemia and its genetic variants. *Journal of Bone and Joint Surgery,* **51A,** 33–57.

Golding J. S. R., McIvor R. & Went L. N. (1959) The bone changes in sickle cell anaemia and its genetic variants. *Journal of Bone and Joint Surgery,* **41B,** 711–8.

Iwegbu C. G. & Fleming A. F. (1985) Avascular necrosis of the femoral head in sickle cell disease. *Journal of Bone and Joint Surgery,* **67B,** 29–32.

Washington E. R. & Root L. (1985) Conservative treatment of sickle cell avascular necrosis of the femoral head. *Journal of Pediatric Orthopedics,* **5,** 192–4.

Leukaemia

Jones P. G., Campbell H. E. & Beardmore H. F. (1976) *Tumours of Infancy and Childhood.* Blackwell Scientific Publications, Oxford.

Lanzkowsky P. (1983) *Pediatric Oncology.* McGraw Hill, New York.

Ragab A. N. Frech R. S. & Vietti J. J. (1970) Osteoporotic fractures secondary to methotrexate therapy of acute leukaemia with remission. *Cancer,* **5,** 580–5.

Rogalsky R. J., Black J. B. & Reed M. H. (1986) Orthopaedic manifesations of leukaemia in children. *Journal of Bone and Joint Surgery,* **68A,** 494–501.

Idiopathic chondrolysis

Duncan J. W., Nasca R. & Schranz J. (1979) Idiopathic chondrolysis of the hip. *Journal of Bone and Joint Surgery,* **61A,** 1024–8.

Jones B. S. (1971) Adolescent chondrolysis of the hip joint. *South African Medical Journal,* **45,** 196–202.

Mankin H., Sledge C., Rothschild S. & Einstein A. (1975) Chondrolysis of the hip. In 'The Hip'. (Ed. Riley L. H. Jr.) Published by C. V. Mosby, St. Louis.

Epiphyseal dysplasias

Crossan J. F. Wynne-Davies R. & Fulford G. E. (1983) Bilateral failure of the capital femoral epiphysis: bilateral Perthes disease, multiple epiphyseal dysplasia, pseudo achondroplasia and spondyloepiphyseal dysplasia congenita and tarda. *Journal of Pediatric Orthopedics,* **3,** 297–301.

Lachmann R. S., Rimion D. L. & Hollister D. W. (1973) Arthrography of the hip: A clue to the pathogenesis of the epiphyseal dysplasias. *Radiology,* **108,** 317–22.

Spranger J. (1976) Epiphyseal dysplasias. *Clinical Orthopedics and Related Research,* **114,** 46–9.

Wynne-Davies R. & Hall C. (1982) Two clinical variants of spondylo epiphyseal dysplasia. *Journal of Bone and Joint Surgery,* **64B,** 435–41.

Synovial osteochondromatosis

McIvor R. R. & King D. (1962) Osteochondromatosis of the hip joint. *Journal of Bone and Joint Surgery,* **44A,** 87–97.

Pelker R. R., Drennan J. C. & Ozomoff M. B. (1983) Juvenile synovial chondromatosis of the hip. *Journal of Bone and Joint Surgery,* **65A,** 552–4.

Milgram J. W. & Pease C. N. (1980) Synovial osteochondromatosis in a young child. *Journal of Bone and Joint Surgery,* **62A,** 1021–3.

Fibrous dysplasia

Funk F. J. & Wells R. E. (1973) Hip problems in fibrous dysplasia. *Clinical Orthopaedics and Related Research,* **90,** 77–82.

Nakashima Y, Kotoura Y., Yamamuro T. & Hamashima Y. (1984) Monostotic fibrous dysplasia in the femoral neck. *Clinical Orthopaedics and Related Research,* **191,** 242–8.

Bone cysts

Campanna R., Dalmonte A., Gitelis S. & Campanacci M. (1982) The natural history of unilateral bone cyst after steroid injection. *Clinical Orthopedics and Related Research,* **166,** 209–11.

Chigira M., Maehara S., Arita S. & Udagawa E. (1983). The aetiology and treatment of simple bone cysts. *Journal of Bone and Joint Surgery,* **65B**, 633–7.

Feller A. M., Thielemann F. & Flach A. (1982) Long term results in the treatment of juvenile bone cysts. *Zeitschrift für kinderchirurgie und Grenzgebiete,* **36**, 138–42.

Malawar *et al.* (1985) Unilateral bone cysts treated by renografin injection and intracavity methyl prednisolone acetate. *Journal of Pediatric Orthopedics,* **5**, 499.

Oppenheim L. & Galleno H. (1984) Operation v's methyl prednisolone acetate in unicameral bone cysts. *Journal of Pediatric Orthopedics,* **4**, 17.

Scaglietti O., Marchetti P. G. & Bartolozzi P. (1979) The effects of methyl prednisolone acetate in the treatment of bone cysts. *Journal of Bone and Joint Surgery,* **61B**, 200–4.

Smith *et al.* (1985). Early results steroid injections in unilateral bone cysts. *Journal of Pediatric Orthopedics,* **5**, 499.

Osteoid osteoma

Colton C. L. & Hardy J. G. (1983) Evaluation of a sterilizable radiation probe as an aid to surgical treatment of osteoid osteoma. *Journal of Bone and Joint Surgery,* **65A**, 1019–22.

Enneking W. F. (1983) *Musculoskeletal Tumor Surgery,* Churchill Livingstone, New York.

Goldberg V. M. & Jacobs B. (1975) Osteoid osteoma of the hip in children. *Clinical Orthopedics and Related Research,* **106**, 41-7.

Golding J. S. R. (1954) The natural history of osteoid osteoma. *Journal of Bone and Joint Surgery,* **36B**, 218–29.

Jackson R. P., Reckling F. W. & Mautz F. A. (1977) Osteoid osteoma and osteoblastoma: similar histological lesions with different natural histories. *Clinical Orthopaedics and Related Research,* **128**, 303–12.

Johnson G. F. (1953) Osteoid osteoma of the femoral neck. *American Journal of Roentgenology,* **74**, 65.

Kumar S. J., Harcke H. T. & McEwen D. G. (1984) Osteoid osteoma of the proximal femur: New techniques in diagnosis and treatment. *Journal of Pediatric Orthopedics,* **4**, 669–72.

Moberg E. (1951) The natural course of osteoid osteoma. *Journal of Bone and Joint Surgery,* **33A**, 166.

Norman A. & Dorfmann H. D. (1975) Osteoid osteoma inducing pronounced overgrowth and deformity of bone. *Clinical Orthopaedics and Related Research,* **110**, 233–8.

Omojola M. F., Cockshatt W. P. & Beatty E. G. (1981) Osteoid osteoma — An evaluation of diagnostic modalities. *Clinical Radiology,* **32**, 199–204.

Sim F. H., Dahlin D. C. & Beabout J. (1975) Osteoid osteoma — Diagnostic problems. *Journal of Bone and Joint Surgery,* **57A**, 154–9.

Spence A. J. & Lloyd-Roberts G. C. (1961) Regional osteoporosis in osteoid osteoma. *Journal of Bone and Joint Surgery,* **43B**, 501–7.

Swee R. G., McLeod R. A. & Beabout J. (1979) Osteoid osteoma. *Radiology,* **30**, 117.

Eosinophilic granuloma

Cohen M., Zornoza J., Zornoza J., Cangir A., Murray J. & Wallace S. (1980). Direct injection of methylprednisolone sodium succinate in the treatment of solitary eosinophilic granuloma. *Radiology,* **136**, 289–93.

Enneking W. F. (1983) *Muskuloskeletal Tumour Surgery,* Churchill Livingstone, New York.

Fowler J. V. & Bobechko W. P. (1970) Solitary eosinophilic granuloma in bone. *Journal of Bone and Joint Surgery,* **52B**, 238–43.

Leeson M. C., Smith A., Carter J. R. & Makley J. T. (1985) Eosinophilic granuloma of bone in the growing epiphysis. *Journal of Pediatric Orthopedics,* **5**, 147–50.

Sartoris D. J. & Parker B. R. (1984) Histiocytosis X — rate and pattern of resolution of osseus lesions. *Radiology,* **152**, 679–84.

Lichtenstein L. (1977) *Bone Tumours,* p. 190. C. V. Mosby & Co, St. Louis.

Lloyd-Roberts G. C. and Ratliffe A. H. (1978). *Hip Disorders in Children,* Butterworths & Co., London.

Secondary Tumours

Lanzkowsky P. (1983) *Pediatric Oncology,* McGraw Hill, New York.

Benign tumours

Enneking W. F. (1983) *Muskuloskeletal Tumor Surgery,* Churchill Livingstone, New York.
Cole W. G. (1986) Treatment of aneurysmal bone cysts in childhood. *Journal of Pediatric Orthopedics,* **6,** 326–9.

Index